Developments in Pre-registration Nursing Education

An International Perspective

Report prepared for The Commission on Nursing

July 1998

By

MARK P. TYRRELL

RGN, RPN, RNT, BNS, MEd

Lecturer, Department of Nursing Studies
National University of Ireland, Cork

Edited by

DR. GERALDINE MC CARTHY-HASLAM

RGN, RNT, MEd, MSN, PhD

Director, Department of Nursing Studies
National University of Ireland, Cork

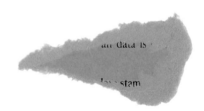

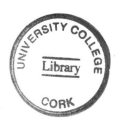

ISBN 0-7076-6131-5

BAILE ÁTHA CLIATH
ARNA FHOILSIÚ AG OIFIG AN tSOLÁTHAIR
Le ceannach díreach ón
OIFIG DHÍOLTA FOILSEACHÁN RIALTAIS,
TEACH SUN ALLIANCE, SRÁID THEACH LAIGHEAN, BAILE ÁTHA CLIATH 2,
nó tríd an bpost ó
FOILSEACHÁIN RIALTAIS, AN RANNÓG POST-TRÁCHTA,
4 - 5 BÓTHAR FHEARCHAIR, BAILE ÁTHA CLIATH 2,
(Teil: 01 - 6613111 – fo-líne 4040/4045; Fax: 01 - 4752760)
nó trí aon díoltóir leabhar.

———————

DUBLIN
PUBLISHED BY THE STATIONERY OFFICE
To be purchased directly from the
GOVERNMENT PUBLICATIONS SALE OFFICE,
SUN ALLIANCE HOUSE, MOLESWORTH STREET, DUBLIN 2,
or by mail order from
GOVERNMENT PUBLICATIONS, POSTAL TRADE SECTION,
4 - 5 HARCOURT ROAD, DUBLIN 2,
(Tel: 01 - 6613111 – ext. 4040/4045; Fax: 01 - 4752760)
or through any bookseller.

———————

£7.00

PREFACE

On March 21st 1997, the Minister for Health, Mr. Michael Noonan, T.D., established the Commission on Nursing. The terms of reference were: to examine and report on the role of nurses in the health service including:

- the evolving role of nurses, reflecting their professional development and the overall management of services;
- promotional opportunities and related difficulties;
- structural and work changes appropriate for the effective and efficient discharge of that role;
- the requirements placed on nurses, both in training and the delivery of services;
- segmentation of the grade;
- training and educational requirements; and
- the role and function of An Bord Altranais generally, including, *inter alia*, education and professional development, regulation and protection of the citizen.

As part of the preparatory work a number of reports were commissioned. This report entitled "Developments in Pre-Registration Nursing Education – An International Perspective" has been prepared by Mark Tyrrell and edited by Dr. Geraldine McCarthy-Haslam.

Ms. Justice Mella Carroll
Chair of the
Commission on Nursing

July 1998

iii

TABLE OF CONTENTS

Chapter 2: Changes in Nurse Education – Australia and New Zealand

LIST OF TABLES

INTRODUCTION

This report represents the results of a literature review that was undertaken on behalf of the Commission on Nursing. The purpose of the review was to critically examine pre-registration nursing education internationally and in doing so, the report focuses specifically on current developments in nurse education in the United Kingdom, Australia, Canada and New Zealand. In particular, the report concentrates on degree level preparation and on the process of merging/linking with third level educational institutions. The type of curriculum models used are identified, and a number of other curricular issues analysed, such as selection of students and the accreditation of programmes. The report also examines the relationships that exist between the colleges and the associated schools of nursing both during and after the merging process. The literature is further examined with regard to the arrangements for students' clinical education and of the funding of nurse education in each of these countries. The outcomes, transition to practice and career paths of graduates from these programmes is then analysed and the implications of the changes for nurse educators are considered.

In Chapter One, current developments in nurse education in the United Kingdom (UK) are considered. An historical perspective of degree level nurse education is given. This is followed by a broad account of Project 2000, the current diploma level pre-registration programme. Consideration is also given to recent trends in the UK towards pre-registration degree level preparation.

The focus of Chapter Two is on recent developments in nurse education in Australia and New Zealand. An account of the transition of nurse education in these two countries to the higher education sector at diploma level is given, and an examination of the subsequent upgrading to degree status is conducted.

Chapter Three considers the developments in nurse education that have taken place in Canada over the past decade. The initial move from hospital-based schools of nursing to diploma programmes in Community Colleges is examined, as is the subsequent move towards the Baccalaureate degree as the sole entry criteria to professional nursing practice.

An overview of nurse education in France is given in Chapter Four. This is necessarily brief due to the lack of literature published in English. Some details of nurse education in other European countries are presented as an Appendix to the report. A summary and conclusion to the report is given thereafter.

CHAPTER 1

CHANGES IN NURSE EDUCATION — THE UNITED KINGDOM

1.1 The Traditional Programme

Traditionally, nurse education in the United Kingdom followed the apprenticeship model whereby student nurses were employed to learn on the job and their educational needs were seen as subordinate to the needs of the service (Dolan, 1993). Logan (1987) suggests that for many years now, the apprenticeship model has been recognised as a system which nullifies any serious attempt to improve the training of nurses. Moreover, Hayward (1982) makes the point that characteristically, the product of an apprenticeship model will know a great deal about a defined area of work and will possess very advanced skills. Knowledge of wider issues in the area, may however, be limited by comparison with a graduate. The author gives the example of a fitter or toolmaker compared to a graduate engineer stating that initially the former may be more proficient at certain skills but in time the graduate engineer will become master of a wide array and skills. The apprentice ship model, which was first established by Nightingale in the 1840s, survived for over one hundred years however, despite many attempts on the part of the profession and other interested parties to change this approach to nurse education and training.

1.2 Developments in Nurse Education in the Higher Education Sector

Developments in Pre-registration Degree Programmes

According to Altschul (1987), the major impetus in forging links with colleges of higher education occurred between 1950 and 1960. Courses for nurse teachers and health visitors lead the way, and shortly afterwards, there followed a number of experimental courses between hospitals and colleges. What is significant about all of these courses however, is that despite their experimental status, all were immediately over subscribed to, and all proved that a pool of able recruits existed, keen to enter nursing if its education programmes were attractively organised (Altschul, 1987).

The UK has a relatively short history of nursing degree programmes (Milligan, 1997). Unlike countries such as Canada and the United States where nursing degree programmes date back to the first quarter of the 20th century, the first pre-registration nursing degree

1

in the UK was instigated in Edinburgh in 1960. At this time however, it is reported that up to 30 percent of all nurses in the United States held either a Bachelors or an Associate degree (Altschul, 1987).

In 1956, a nursing studies unit was established at the University of Edinburgh. Two years later, the first pre-registration degree course commenced in conjunction with a number of local hospitals and health service agencies, leading to a BSc social science-nursing degree, registration as a general nurse, and a national district nursing certificate (Montague and Herbert, 1982). While the medical faculty at the college expressed interest in the course during early negotiations, it subsequently did not accept the course. The faculty of Arts did accept it however, but would not recognise the nursing studies courses as part fulfilment of its degree requirements (Altschul, 1987). A similar degree was offered at Manchester University in 1969. Graduates with this degree also qualify for general nurse registration and obtain a district nursing and health visiting certificate (Montague and Herbert, 1982). There followed a number of similar programmes in other universities including those at Hull and Surrey (Kemp, 1988). It would appear that by 1987, there were over 20 such degree programmes available throughout the UK (Howard and Brooking, 1987). These degree programmes were run in tandem with the traditional pre-registration nurse education programmes.

Outcomes of These Early Under-graduate Programmes

A number of outcome studies have been carried out by university departments of nursing offering degrees to nurses, the aim of which were to examine the career paths of graduates (Kemp, 1988; Bircumshaw and Chapman, 1988; Reid, et al., 1987; Howard and Brooking, 1987; Montague and Herbert, 1982 and, Marsh, 1976). Milligan (1997) reports that response rates in all of these studies ranged from 75% to 100%, with sample sizes ranging from 48 in the Howard and Brooking (1987) study to 100 in the Montague and Herbert (1982) study, thus giving an average sample size of 80.4 participants per study.

Myths about graduate nurses abound in the literature. These include: the myth of non entry to nursing; the myth of rapid promotion; the myth of non-stickability and, the myth of non-clinical involvement (Sinclair, 1987). Sinclair draws attention to the fact that while no one knows the number of nurse graduates in the UK, their careers have been the subject of an inordinate amount of speculation and research. Most of the outcome studies take the form of a retrospective annual questionnaire (Milligan, 1997), and most agree that the vast majority of graduates from these programmes enter clinical practice on qualifying, and indeed remain in clinical practice just as long as traditionally prepared nurses (MacGuire, 1991). The author proposes that there is scant evidence to suggest that these nurses are fast-tracked to more lucrative career paths. Indeed, an analysis of the findings of the studies clearly lays to rest a number of myths that prevail regarding the career paths of these graduates.

The Myth of Non Entry to Nursing

Milligan (1997), in a review of a number of key studies of career paths of nurse graduates (Bircumshaw and Chapman, 1988a, 1988b; Howard and Brooking, 1987; Kemp, 1988; Montague and Herbert, 1982; Reid et al., 1987; Sinclair, 1984, and Scott-Wright et al., 1979) points out that on average, over 90% of these nurses immediately enter clinical nursing practice after graduation. For example, Reid, et al., (1987), report that 96% of respondents were in clinical posts after graduation, while Sinclair (1984) points out that :

Each year, on average, at least 93% of these respondents remain employed, almost all of them on nursing and mainly clinical posts in hospital. Even if it is assumed that all non-respondents have left nursing (and this is almost certainly not the case), then 80% of graduates are nursing during the two years following completion of the degree programme (Sinclair, 1984, p. 56).

Such findings are echoed by most of the other evaluators of the early degree programmes. For example, Howard and Brooking report that 77% of respondents were in nursing posts two years after qualifying, while the figures for the Montague and Herbert (1982) and the Bircumshaw and Chapman (1988) studies are 67.5% and 93% respectively. However, there is some evidence that nurses who subsequently become graduates do not remain in nursing. For instance, MacGuire and Sparks (1970) found that there was a correlation between graduating after qualifying as a nurse and moving out of nursing after graduation.

The Myth of Rapid Promotion

Sinclair (1987) asserts that one of the most persistent beliefs about nurse graduates is that they are fast-tracked to promotion, particularly into management posts. Evidence from the outcome studies show that this is indeed far from the truth, so much so that Professor Altschul (1983) publicly lamented this group's lack of ambition and career aspirations to move into senior nursing posts. In Sinclair's (1982) study, only 3 out of 189 respondents were working at nursing officer grade, and Reid and colleagues report from Northern Ireland that:

> ...striking that not a single respondent indicated an aspiration to move into nursing administration, and that half intended to stay in clinical practice with the remainder mostly aiming at nursing education (Reid et al., 1987, p.222).

Milligan (1997) points out that this lack of movement into management posts is somewhat of a cause for celebration for these researchers as it demonstrates that graduate nurses are not too academic to survive in clinical practice, and perhaps also, that they therefore might represent more value for money than expected.

While the criteria used to define senior posts or nursing administration in these studies is not always clear, it would appear that most senior posts seem to have been at ward sister, and nurse specialist level. Furthermore, it is also evident from this research that many nurses pursue additional studies both within and without nursing, (Reid et al., 1987; Sinclair, 1985; Montague and Herbert, 1982), the majority doing so within 3 years of graduation.

The Myth of Non-Stickability

This myth alleges that even if nurse graduates do enter clinical nursing, the majority will not remain. Again, the overwhelming evidence is that this is not the case. Scott - Wright and associates report how at each year's follow up of their cohort of graduates, between 70% and 75% were in nursing posts. Similarly, Sinclair (1984), at the five year follow up found that 68% of respondents were still in nursing posts, while Bircumshaw and Chapman (188) cited almost 72% as still working in nursing posts after five years. Indeed, Sinclair reports that over 60% of graduates were in nursing ten years after graduation, almost one fifth of whom were in hospital posts (Sinclair, 1984). These figures compare favourably with the expected length of service contribution of traditionally trained nurses which is estimated to be 5-7 years on average in Northern Ireland (Reid, 1986).

An analysis of why graduates leave nursing shows that the vast majority do so due to pregnancy and childrearing (Kemp, 1988; Reid et al., 1987; Sinclair, 1987 and Montague and Herbert, 1982). Moreover, when asked if they intended to return to nursing, over two thirds of respondents in Kemp's (1988) study answered in the affirmative. A significant minority of these graduates however, tend to leave nursing as a result of frustration with their role as a nurse or due to general dissatisfaction with the job. Montague and Herbert (1982, p.368) report that seven of the 100 respondents in their study left as a result of finding "no academic stimulus" in the job, while four respondents cited "rigid attitudes within the profession" as their reason for leaving. Other reasons for leaving (besides motherhood) were no job satisfaction (n=1), no career prospects (n=1), poor pay (n=3), and unsocial hours (n=2).

The Myth of Non-Clinical Involvement

It is evident from these studies that clinical nursing posts remain popular among nurse graduates even after five years. In particular, these studies demonstrate a predilection among graduates for posts in the community, in midwifery, and also as clinical specialists (Bircumshaw and Chapman, 1988; Sinclair, 1987 and, Montague and Herbert, 1982). Sinclair (1984) comments that this move towards specialist posts can only serve to benefit the profession in the future. With regard to the tendency of these graduates to move towards community posts, Milligan (1997) notes that is has been common for the degree programmes to be associated with community related qualifications. For example, the degree programme held at Manchester university between 1969 and 1972 lead not only to a degree in nursing, but also to registration as a general nurse, and qualifications in district nursing and Health visiting. Furthermore, one of the most popular areas for further study of these graduates was health visiting (Milligan, 1997). While it is therefore not unusual for a trend towards community nursing to occur, it is arguable that these graduates move to such posts as a result of the autonomy accorded to nurses working in areas such as community, midwifery and clinical specialisms. Clearly this is an issue that needs further study. Also, this trend towards community is one that should be encouraged given recent trends in health provision with an emphasis on primary health care (WHO 1985, Department of Health, 1994).

While a clear majority of graduates profiled in the outcome studies remained in clinical nursing, a significant minority moved into research and education posts. However, these are not always posts which are directly related to nursing (Milligan, 1997). It can be seen from this evidence that despite the myths, the majority of graduate nurses from the early degree programmes enter clinical nursing posts upon graduation, are not fast-tracked to senior posts, and very much remain at the patients bedside. Sinclair, (1987) concludes that these nurses appear to be setting their sights lower than their real potential might justify, suggesting that this might be as a result of the very myths outlined. The author urges better career guidance and encouragement for these nurses.

While, et al., (1995) conducted a substantial piece of research that was commissioned by the English National Board, the focus of which was to compare the outcomes of pre-registration nurse education programmes. The researchers using a triangulation research design that incorporated participant and non-participant observation, video taped simulations, and care planning exercises, studied the differences between nurses from

RGN programmes (n=34), Project 2000 diploma programmes (n=34) and Integrated RGN degree programmes (n=31). The authors acknowledge that a larger sample would have increased the generalisability of the findings, however, this was not possible due to the fact that so few students were undertaking degree programmes. The findings suggest that the degree students scored highest on care planning and more of these students espoused a client focus rather than a professional focus to their practice. Further, this group valued more the contribution of their teachers during the programme. The Project 2000 students on the other hand identified skills as an area of perceived confidence deficit and suggested continued learning in the practice setting and more clinical placements as potential strategies for overcoming such deficits. The RGN students demonstrated their extensive clinical practice base and were much influenced by their greater clinical exposure. Further, this group made significantly more requests for clarification of the nurses role. The researchers point out that the similarities of this group and the Project 2000 group was most evident in the observational data however, in certain domains of nursing practice there was a trend indicating that the RGN group were more able to demonstrate skills. Both the RGN group and the Project 2000 group suggested that their courses of study required some modification. The authors concluded that the corresponding performance scores of the RGN and Project 2000 programmes is remarkable, however, there was a steady trend regarding the cogency of the integrated degree programme in providing a sound foundation for nursing practice (While et al, 1995).

Milligan (1997), having reviewed these key studies, points out that the similarity of methods used is both a strength and a weakness. Their strength lies in the fact that the researchers have presented a reasonably clear picture about the career patterns of nurse graduates from the programmes. A limitation of the studies however, is that with the changing context of health care, nurse education and clinical practice, the findings only tentatively inform the reader as to what pattern newer graduates may take. Furthermore, Fitzpatrick et al., (1993) urge caution in interpreting outcome studies as they say very little, if anything, about the clinical performance of the graduates concerned. Milligan also challenges the researchers for omitting to compare nurse graduates with nurses who were prepared for practice through non-graduate routes (Milligan, 1997).

Recent Links with Third Level

Over the last decade or so, links between nurse education and the higher education sector have continued to develop both as a result of the implementation of Project 2000, and also as a result of the increasing number of pre-registration degree programmes that are being offered by colleges of nursing and midwifery in collaboration with institutes of higher education. In this section, the main catalysts involved in these developments are discussed, and the implications of such links for all concerned are analysed.

Traditionally, colleges of nursing and midwifery have had close links with district health authorities, which provided them with premises and administration support, and funded student nurses salaries. With the separation of purchasers and providers under the new National HealthService (NHS) reforms however, the management of training institutions became secondary to the districts' key responsibilities, namely, the identification of health needs of the community and the purchase of health care to meet those needs (National Audit Office [NAO], 1992). As a result of this, the Department of Health undertook a review of the status and management of the colleges and considered it likely that closer links with the higher education sector would be developed (Department of Health, 1989).

At about the same time (1987), the initial proposals for project 2000 were published. Curricula for traditional nurse education programmes were developed locally by individual colleges in line with guidelines issued from the National Boards. Such programmes were then submitted to the relevant National Board for validation (Burnard and Chapman, 1990). One of the key aims of the Project 2000 proposals however, was that nursing courses would be given full academic recognition as well as professional recognition (United Kingdom Central Council for Nurses, Midwifery and Health Visiting [UKCC], 1986). The implications of this recommendation therefore, was that stronger links would have to be developed between nurse education and higher education colleges (Bentley, 1996).

The above factors helped to set the scene for further developments in links with higher education, however, evidence is that these links varied considerable in their nature and extent, and were not wholly successful in all cases (Jowett, et al., 1994).

In 1994, Jowett et al., published a final report of their study on the implementation of Project 2000. The study, funded by the Department of Health, was carried out over a period of three years in six of the 13 first round Demonstration sites in England- (those that started the diploma course in late 1989 or early 1990), and entailed interviews with a sample of all of the key players involved in the programme (students, nurse teachers, staff from higher education (HE), nurse managers, and clinical nurses) at a number of points in time over the three years. The authors report a variety of links having developed over the duration of the study. Some colleges of nursing had advanced towards full integration with the HE institution to which they were linked. Two were established as schools of nursing within the HE faculty structure with a newly appointed head from a nurse education background, whilst another had become an institute within the link institution of Higher Education. At least one college of nursing however, was preparing to split from their third level link institution and develop another affiliation with a different college. In another situation, the only role of the higher education link institution was to validate the nursing programme. In this latter case there was no student contact with HE, however, staff from both institutions worked together on a number of committees involving curriculum development, examinations, and academic standards. In another case, amalgamation of the college of nursing with its link institution was to take place whereby it was to become a department within the HE institution.

Much of the early (and in some cases ongoing) difficulties regarding these links seem to have resulted from differing expectations of the relationship on the part of the two institutions, namely, the college of nursing and the third level institution, and perhaps also an element of ignorance regarding the other's culture, traditions and purposes. For example, Jowett et al., (1994) report how in one institution, a senior member of HE staff closely involved in the link, described it as a "nightmare" (p.23) and reported serious misunderstandings over organisational and structural relations between the two parties involved. It would also appear from the report that there was much mistrust on the part of HE staff, and also, concern was expressed that staff at the college of nursing were planning to go it alone. Indeed the authors suggest that in fact this may well have been the case in at least one instance whereby staff at one college of nursing expressed the wish to split from HE within four to five years. Similarly, nurse educators also had feelings of mistrust. In particular, concerns were expressed at what was perceived to be the imminent assimilation and control over nursing education by higher education (Henry and Pashley, 1989). A view was also expressed that HE staff did not view their nurse teacher colleagues on an equal footing, particularly in regard to their academic credentials. In this regard, one respondent in Payne et al's (1991) study remarked that "the teachers aren't here teaching – there all out at college just to get more standing in the eyes of the poly!" (p.11). Another possible implication of this situation was that as historically nurse teachers worked in colleges of nursing with a very different ethos to academic disciplines in third level institutions, they had no insights into the roles and functions of institutes of higher education, nor indeed of academic life itself (Charlwood, 1993). This, plus the recommendation of the ENB (1989), that all nurse teachers should have degree level qualifications, placed extra pressure on nurse educators in this time of great change as they juggled with their new roles in HE, tried to cope with the mergers of small colleges of nursing into larger ones, planned the new curriculum and, at the same time read for degrees (Bentley, 1996).

Another disconcerting factor seems to have been the speed at which the programme was implemented. The National Audit Office (1992) report how in many cases approved schemes had received less than six months notice of their starting date. One respondent in Payne et al(1991) study described planning for Project 2000 as being like "laying the lines while the train is coming," and others described it as "ridiculous." (p.1). Many nurse teachers still had commitments to other programmes in terms of teaching and planning, and hence found themselves completely overworked when curriculum planning started in earnest. The result of this was that staff frequently worked late, became over stressed, felt that they were unable to make adequate submissions to curriculum planning, and perhaps most of all at least in some cases, did not collaborate appropriately with their partners in HE to the extent that they would have wished (Payne et al., 1991).

There were also reports of early successes. Many of these can be attributed to the extent of joint communication and collaboration in planning that took place prior to the link. In many of these cases, it emerges that previous joint enterprises had occurred and hence there was much mutual trust established. For example, in one situation a group of four very senior staff (two from each institution), had "collaborated for some considerable time" before the course began (Jowett et al., 1994, p.23). Reciprocal teaching arrangements existed between other institutions, and another report described how a member of HE staff had been seconded part-time to assist the college of nursing with work on the curriculum (Payne et al., 1991).

There have also been a number of recent new pre-registration degree programmes, however, the literature on these programmes is indeed sparse (Milligan, 1997) hence information relating to these programmes will not be dealt with separately, rather it will be interspersed with the discourse on Project 2000.

1.3. Project 2000

The Historical Context of Project 2000

According to Dolan (1993), the seeds for Project 2000 were sown, perhaps as far back as 1943 when a report that was commissioned by the Royal College of Nursing, the Horder Report (RCN, 1943), proposed that the education of nurses should be separated from the needs of service, and that the student nurse be accorded full student status. Unfortunately, these proposals were not acted on by the government of the day and hence little changed with regard to the educational preparation of nurses. In 1947, a government report on the recruitment and training of nurses (Ministry of Health [Wood Report], 1947) called for significant changes to nurse education including full student status and supernumerary status during clinical training. The committee further argued that courses of training should be dictated by the learning needs of the student rather than by the staffing needs of the hospital and consequently, that nurse education should be conducted under the jurisdiction of the training authority rather than the hospital matron. This committee was given a free hand to reconstruct nursing services at a time when plans were being formulated to set up the new NHS (Bentley, 1996). Ironically but perhaps not surprisingly, the proposals were thwarted by the nursing profession itself, most notably the General Nursing Council (GNC) and the RCN, whose ruling councils were dominated by matrons with the vested interests of maintaining their power base, and most of all, of protecting a traditional source of cheap labour (Naish, 1993).

Almost twenty years later, another RCN report, (Platt Report, 1964) was published. Its recommendations were reminiscent of those of the Wood Report (1947) in that the Platt committee argued that a reconstruction of the nurse education system was essential if it were to meet the requirements of the future health needs of the nation, and that the current system of nurse preparation was neither in the best interests of patients, nor of student nurses. The committee emphasised that student nurse training should be grounded in sound educational principles and further recommended that students should be financially independent of the hospital service. As was the case with previous reports, the Platt Report fell foul of some influential nurses, notably matrons and other nurse managers who were concerned primarily about staffing the wards rather than the educational needs of students (Clay, 1987). Needless to say therefore, the report was not implemented. Another probable confounding factor contributing to the rejection of the findings of these key reports was what Altschul (1987) termed the " anti-educational and anti-intellectual stance" commonly encountered in medical and nursing circles, the main thesis of which is that "nursing is a simple job which can be satisfactorily carried out under the instruction and supervision of doctors and that all that should be required of nurses is kindness and a willingness to work hard for long hours and little pay." (p.11).

Over the next decade or so, a number of other reports made some reference to or recommendations for nurse education. It would appear however that these reports made little or no impact on nursing or government policy (Dolan, 1993). Then, in 1972, at a time of considerable industrial unrest in many parts of the British workforce including nursing, a committee was set up under the chairmanship of Professor Asa Briggs to review the work of nurses and midwives, and in particular, to consider educational and training requirements (Bentley, 1996). One of the fundamental problems identified by this committee was the dual and conflicting roles of the student nurse, namely those of learner and worker. Unlike its predecessors, the Briggs committee recommended major policy changes which were to have a very influential effect on the organisation of nursing. In particular, the committee proposed a new statutory framework for nursing, something which Clay (1987) argues placed nursing on a more professional footing thus opening the door for educational reform. The committee also recommended the establishment of colleges of nursing and midwifery, thus paving the way for later merging with higher education. A proposal for a radical change in the organisation of nurse education whereby all prospective nurses and midwives would follow one common basic eighteen month course leading to the award of Certificate in Nursing Practice, was rejected. This common course was to be followed by a further eighteen months of study leading to registration. While the overall report was virtually ignored, many of its features were to re emerge later in the proposals for Project 2000 (Bentley, 1996).

Perhaps the most pertinent and forward thinking of all of the reports into nurse education was that of the committee established in 1978 by the DHSS to re-examine the status of the nurse learner (Bentley, 1996). Of greatest concern to this committee was the ever widening theory-practice gap between nurse education and practice, and the need to ensure that there were enough adequately prepared qualified staff in clinical areas to supervise student's clinical practice. However, no alterations were proposed for nurse training at this stage primarily due to the fact that the statutory changes necessary to establish the UKCC were being planned at the time, but also because policy makers were reticent to alter anything because of the huge financial and manpower implications of moving from an apprenticeship system to a system whereby student nurses would have equal status with other students in higher education (Bentley, 1996).

Background to Project 2000

Notwithstanding the important role that the aforementioned reports played in preparing the groundwork for Project 2000, two documents, which were published on the future of nurse education in 1985, finally cleared the way for the UKCCs 1986 launch of the Project 2000 proposals. The first of these reports (ENB, 1985) examined curriculum content and educational objectives, and recommended that all nurse teachers should be graduates- a move that Bentley (1996) argues was a critical step towards the policy of integrating nurse education with higher education and of securing a more academic preparation for nursing students. The second report, that of the Judge Committee (1985), recommended that nurse education should be separated from the direct and persistent control of service by moving completely into the tertiary education sector, and that students should no longer be employees. Although the recommendation to move nurse education into higher education was not included in the 1986 proposals, this is now taking place with the planned merger of colleges of nursing and institutes of higher education (Bentley, 1996).

In 1986, the UKCC, in association with the four National Boards for nursing, midwifery, and health visiting (England, Scotland, Wales and Northern Ireland), published its proposals for radical changes in the preparation of nurses for practice. The document, entitled *Project 2000: A New Preparation for Practice*, was the result of an extensive consultative process whereby the working group which was established by the Council, consulted widely with the profession by conducting road shows, issuing information papers, and by seeking representations from members from all disciplines within the profession. The UKCC also engaged a firm of management consultants (Price Waterhouse) whose remit was to collect information on manpower requirements, and recruitment and attrition (Burnard and Chapman, (1990). The Council considered that the new education programme, known as Project 2000, would help the NHS address a number of important issues that were currently requiring attention such as, the need to reorient the health services towards illness prevention, the prospect of a marked decrease in the number of recruits to the profession from traditional sources, and the ever increasing need to ensure that services are cost-effective and that they give value for money (NAO, 1992). Whilst acknowledging that the new proposals would be more costly than the traditional system of nurse education, particularly in regard to its initial implementation, the UKCC (1987) outlined a number of both quantifiable and un quantifiable potential benefits to the new programme. Quantifiable benefits included a rationalisation of the current pre-registration programme leading to reduced costs, a reduction in attrition rates of student and qualified nurses, and greater productivity of nurses educated under Project 2000. Other significant expected benefits included an increase in the quality of care, better staff morale which would encourage recruitment and retention, and a flexible workforce capable of adapting to health service needs (NAO, 1992).

The final recommendations were presented to the Government for consideration. In doing so, the Department carried out its own estimation of the likely costs and concluded that the additional costs would amount to £580 million over fourteen years, at 1987 prices, and assuming that Project 2000 was introduced over a ten year period (NAO, 1992).

In 1988, the Department of Health declared its broad acceptance of the UKCCs (1987) proposals (with some modifications). These proposals are outlined in Table 1.1.

TABLE 1.1. The Project 2000 Proposals

— Nursing education would consist of an 18 month common foundation programme followed by a further 18 months in one of the four branch programmes- adult, child, mental health, and mental handicap nursing.[1]

— Greater emphasis would be placed on Health Promotion in the new curriculum.

— Student nurses would no longer be part of the workforce, rather, that they would have student status with non means-tested bursaries instead of salaries.

— While the amount of time that students would be rostered for duty on wards would be substantially reduced, their education would remain practical and patient oriented.[2]

— There would be a wider range of placements with more emphasis on experience of health care in community settings.

— Nursing education would develop close links with higher education, and that on completion of the new course, in addition to nurse registration, students would receive a qualification of, at least, a diploma in higher education.

— Nursing education should lead to only one level of registered nurse, and hence the abolition of the enrolled nurse grade, a grade which had been in place since the end of World War Two.

— Education programmes should be made available to enrolled nurses to enable them to convert to registered nurse status.

[1] The initial proposal included midwifery as a fifth branch, however, this lead to objections from a number of quarters, most notably from the midwifery profession itself who had its own plans for the future education of its students (Burnard and Chapman, 1990).

[2] Students were to be rostered for ward duties for a period of 18 weeks in their final year in preparation for professional practice.

Source: **UKCC,** *Project 2000: The Final Proposals* – **Project Paper No. 9. 1989.**

Goals of Project 2000

The ultimate goals of the Project 2000 proposals were according to Robinson, (1991) an attempt to increase the professional status of nurses with respect to other health care professionals, and further, to enhance nurses' acquisition of the skills required for autonomous practice. A further goal of the new curriculum according to Casey (1996), was to prepare nurses to meet the changing health care requirements of future populations. Moreover, Chandler (1991) describes Project 2000 as an education system which would provide enhanced autonomy and quality in practice, enhanced nursing research capabilities, a redefined role for nursing, and, a wider pool of recruits. This latter aspect was deemed particularly important due to the projected shortage of suitably qualified female school leavers (the traditional recruit for a career in nursing), to fill the number of places required by the profession (NAO, 1992).

Practical and Philosophical Underpinnings of the Project 2000 Curriculum

The following is a summary of Jowett et al's (1994) overview of the broad philosophical underpinnings of the Project 2000 curriculum. Other issues concerning the curriculum are discussed in different sections of this chapter.

Project 2000 is a major innovation in the educational preparation of student nurses for registration as nurses. It is comprised of a common foundation of 18 months duration, followed by a further 18 month's branch in one of the nursing specialities, general nursing, mental nursing, sick children's nursing, or mental handicap nursing. Other aspects of the programme include increased links with higher education, supernumerary status for students (except for a short period of rostered paid clinical practice in the final year), payment by means of bursaries, and the award of a diploma on successful completion of the programme. The entry requirement's for nurse education (and the principle of a wider gate of entry), did not change when Project 2000 was introduced.

According to Jowett et al (1994), while the principles and aims of Project 2000 have been variously interpreted in practice, there are some common grounds. A plethora of words and phrases have been associated with the programme, such as holistic care, client/patient centred care, student centred learning, communication, research based practice, knowledgeable doer, and accountability. The desired outcomes of the diplomate are identified by Jowett et al (1994) as follows:
The diplomate should be able to:

- critically analyse and synthesise material and engage in cogent argument;

- understand the research process and be critical of research methodology and findings that may be applied in practice;

- explain and justify practice that is based on a thorough theoretical grounding and the application of research, to their peers and a multidisciplinary team;

- practice autonomously;

- demonstrate professional accountability and commitment to continuing professional education and development;

- give safe, compassionate, competent nursing care which acknowledges the individuality, stage of development and rights of the adult and is based on a model of nursing;

- demonstrate competence and confidence in communication and teaching of adults, families and colleagues;

- assign appropriate work to helpers and provide supervision and monitoring of assigned work.

The major educational philosophical stance of Project 2000 is one of student centredness which is mirrored in the holistic approach to patient care, and also on combining a series of subjects into a nursing course. While the curriculum is nursing lead, it is underpinned by a foundation in the biological and behavioural sciences as well as in an appreciation of the research process. Moreover, the course is designed to facilitate the development of lifelong learning.

Students are rostered for clinical placement in the Branch Programme for 20% of their time and a wide variety of placements are offered in terms of location, duration, and client group. Clinical experiences generally progress from a *well client* focus at the start of the Common Foundation Programme (CFP), towards an *ill client* focus at the end of the Branch Programme. In some sites, students have little or no contact with hospitals in their CFP, while in others, students have short hospital placements in the first term. Community placements are similarly varied, some place an emphasis on having students placed in shops, factories and industry.

Great emphasis is placed in the curriculum on a health focus and on the inherent dignity and value of the client in line with the humanistic philosophy of the programme. A significant feature of the clinical practice component is on the provision of non-institutional and community based placements in an effort to produce a practitioner who can function in institutional settings as well as in the community.

Each college develops its own curriculum along these broad philosophical guidelines, and hence the course on each site offers differing combinations of the physical and social sciences interwoven with practice placements. While the CFP usually contains a wide variety of community and hospital placements, the emphasis in the Branch Programmes in on institutional placements and on relevant academic work. Overall, 50% of the programmes comprises the academic component, and 50% the practice component. For example, a breakdown from one site (Adult Branch) of a standard 2,300 hours programme, is 950 hours of the art and science of nursing (largely placements and time for reflection); 500 hours on the development and function of the individual (including microbiology and pharmacology); 500 hours on the individual and society (including psychology in nursing) and 350 hours on ethics and politics in relation to nursing (including nursing management).

With regard to who teaches what, and where, Jowett et al (1994) report from the demonstration districts that Higher Education's' staff teaching input in the first common foundation programmes varies. In one of the sites evaluated, HE staff taught biology only, whereas in another they taught social science, biological science, information technology, and management. The norm was for HE staff to teach most if not all of these sciences. Similarly, there was great diversity in the locations for HE staff input. For example, in some sites students spent one day per week at the HE institution, while at others all course teaching, including nursing, was carried out at the HE site. Recently, there has been further amalgamation of former colleges of nursing into HE institutions, indeed, many have completely merged at this point in time. Hence much more of the teaching is conducted at the HE institution. A detailed and lengthy description of the key features of the demonstration districts is available as an appendix in Jowett et al's (1994) report.

1.4 Funding of Nurse Education

Background

Nurses are the main providers of direct patient care in most Western countries and this is also the case in the National Health Service in the United Kingdom. The NHS nursing workforce in England, (including midwives, health visitors, auxiliary nurses, and student nurses), numbers over 400,000 staff and their wage bill expenditure amounts to over £5 billion per annum. This represents about 20% of total expenditure on the health programme. On average, about 20,000 nurses are required each year to replace those who retire or who leave the service for other reasons and in 1992 the National Audit Office reported that there were about 50,000 student nurses undergoing pre-registration training in the NHS at an estimated cost of over £600 million per annum (NAO, 1992). Traditionally, as well as approving educational institutions and nursing courses, the National Boards paid the salaries of over 5000 college staff while the NHS owned and managed most colleges, and funded students' salaries or bursaries (NAO, 1992). In 1993, these arrangements changed in an effort to simplify the financing of nurse education and to secure better value for money for the estimated £600 million spent on pre-registration nursing education each year. Since April 1993, regional health authorities have had sole responsibility for financing nursing education, instead of sharing this responsibility with the National Boards. Regions estimate their student nurse requirements in consultation with employers and purchase training from colleges under contract. It was felt that this should clarify the costs of training, assist employers in determining how best to meet demand for qualified nursing staff, and meet their requirements for student nurses (NAO, 1992).

Financing Project 2000

In the mid 1980s, the UKCC in conjunction with the four National Boards, developed Project 2000, and in doing so, commissioned a detailed analysis of the programmes projected financial costs. Estimates were that Project 2000 would increase the cost of training each student nurse by 25% (UKCC, 1987). While it was expected that savings would be made by providing students with a bursary instead of a salary, extra costs would be incurred by increased educational provision, and by having to replace student labour. (In the traditional programme, student nurses contributed significantly towards the overall nursing labour force). The UKCC argued however, that because the Project 2000 nurse would be better prepared and hence more effective and efficient, and that less wastage would occur due to the expected attractiveness of the new course, training costs would be reduced by the year 2004 (Bentley, 1996).

After receiving the UKCCs proposals for Project 2000 (UKCC, 1987), the Department of Health undertook its own cost analysis and concluded that the extra education and service costs associated with Project 2000 would amount to £580 million over 14 years, that is assuming that the programme was introduced over a ten year period (NAO, 1992). One of the main reasons identified for the considerable increase in costs was that health authorities would need to employ staff to replace their traditional cheap source of labour, namely, student nurses (Dolan, 1993).

In 1989, the Department of Health published the NHS Review White Paper proposing reforms in the funding of the Health Services. Understandably, this raised many concerns regarding the continued implementation of Project 2000 (Payne et al., 1991). However, after raising these concerns with the minister, the profession was given assurances that "whatever arrangements are put in place, the position of nursing, health visiting and midwifery education will be safeguarded.....regard will be taken of the need to maintain the momentum in implementing Project 2000,...[and] the Statutory Bodies will be fully involved in the work." (Burnard and Chapman, 1990, p. 127). Further assurance was given when it was announced by the Department that Project 2000 funding was to be ringfenced. While health authorities can exercise a degree of flexibility in allocating funds between Project 2000 expenditure heads, they cannot spend the funds on other activities. Unspent funds in any one year are carried over to the next. Furthermore, while the Department does not require regions to provide financial reports, the National Boards do (NAO, 1992). The National Audit Office (1992) state however, that some problems have arisen in these accounting procedures. By 1992, few schemes had monitoring systems in place, and finance staff in some schemes complain that it is very difficult, time-consuming and inefficient to maintain separate records for this purpose (NAO, 1992).

Funding at a Central Level – The Department of Health Formula

The costs of replacing the traditional student workforce has been funded at a local level by the Department of Health. After the launch of Project 2000, Health authorities were invited by the Department to submit for funding, and in doing so, were assisted by a set of guidelines set down by the Department's national "Project 2000 Implementation Group". This was one of two groups established at the outset by the Department to oversee the implementation of the Project. The role of this group was to "provide advice and guidance to health authorities, to advise the Department on the feasibility of implementation plans, and to ensure that the agreed timetable was adhered to" (NAO, 1992,p. 11). The second group, the "Steering Group," met only once. Its role was to "agree the continuing timetable, to provide policy guidance, to oversee the work of the Implementation Group and to ensure that common advice and guidance were given to those implementing Project 2000 at the local level" (NAO, 1992,p. 11). In practice it would appear that the Implementation Group have undertaken most of the work associated with the initial implementation of Project 2000.

In providing funding for replacement staff, the Department pointed out that:

> Replacement staff should be identified by grade. There is no formula for this, but the group will challenge any submissions which fall outside a costing parameter of 50% on Scale A [Health care Assistants and Support Workers] and 50% on Scale D [registered nurses]. Within this, a wide variety of combinations of grades are possible and it is open to authorities to reduce the number of replacement staff they require in order to enrich skill mix. For HCA/support workers, the current grading definitions for Scales A and B will continue to apply; an abnormally high proportion of scale B's among replacement staff will be challenged (Department of Health, 1989, para 16).

The principles for replacing student labour as outlined by the Department are outlined in Table 1.2.

TABLE 1.2.   Principles for replacing student labour in Project 2000

- The number of traditional student nurses to be replaced.

- Health authorities were told to estimate that traditional student nurses gave no more than a 60% service contribution (40% in the case of Mental Nursing students).[1]

- Project 2000 students are presently rostered for a service contribution in the final year of the programme equivalent to 50% of that year's total effort . This equates to 20% of the three year course compared with an estimated 60% for general students undertaking traditional nurse training. The service contribution of the traditional students to be replaced therefore consists of the difference between the service contribution lost as a result of the cessation of the old style training, balanced against the service contribution of those undertaking the Project 2000 training. The fact that Project 2000 students only give a service contribution in their final year means that there is no service contribution for the first two years' intakes of these students.

- The service contribution of both traditional and Project 2000 students (expressed in whole time equivalents as per the Departments request), does not take annual leave into account. Therefore, an addition of 10% to the number of replacement staff required was recommended.

- The Department considered that replacement staff (i.e.: registered nurses) would be more efficient than student nurses. They therefore recommended a 20% reduction in the number of replacement staff needed. This was based on the assumption that replacement staff would be permanent and not constantly rotating through placements like students, and that such rotation entailed a degree of inefficiency as a result of the high turnover of students, the need for constant retraining, and the need to rely on relatively inexperienced staff.

- The Department considered that Project 2000 students would be less efficient than traditional students and hence they suggested that Project 2000 student contribution should be reduced by 20% to reflect their presumed lower efficiency.

---

[1] It was emphasised by the Department that the contribution of students who were supernumerary, for example psychiatric placements for general nursing students, could not be included here.

Source adapted from: **Elkan, Hillman and Robinson, *The Implementation of Project 2000 in a District Health Authority,* 1993.**

The National Audit Office (1992) outline how there was much variation in approved costs of the different demonstration schemes over the first five years of the programme. The range of costs was from £1.9 million to £12.8 million, reflecting the size of individual schemes. They also report some of the difficulties that the Implementation Group faced in trying to make meaningful cost comparisons between submissions. Much of these were due to the fundamental differences between schemes. In particular, the Group reported how their consultants had advised them that the cost per student of introducing Project 2000 could justifiably vary by a factor of up to 60% as each scheme was starting from a different funding base (NAO, 1992).

Once college proposals have achieved educational validation from the National Boards and from the HE institutes, the Department of Health allocates the Project 2000 funds (as recommended by the Implementation Group), to the Regional Health Authority to cover the additional service costs, and to the National Board to cover the additional educational costs (NAO, 1992). The method of fund allocation within regions also varies. In general, regions apportion funds to the district health authorities in line with the approved bid. They in turn allocate funds to the colleges, units and trusts involved in the scheme to meet their extra costs (NAO, 1992).

Project 2000 was proving to be more costly than had been anticipated and in July, 1991, following advice from the Implementation Group, the Department made available additional funding of £5 million. The group recommended that these funds be allocated to existing schemes on a pro-rata basis, as it believed that needs were best determined locally (NAO, 1992). However, by November 1991, only one in three regions had passed these funds on to colleges.

Problems with the Formula

These were very much uncharted waters. The changes that Project 2000 brought about were unprecedented. Indeed it has been suggested that any government department could learn much from analysing the magnitude and complexity of the change(NAO, 1992). As a result, many of the components of the Department's formula were based on unproved assumptions and the complexity of the overall funding arrangements lead to some variation in interpretation. Not surprisingly therefore, difficulties arose in their operationalisation. For instance, the National Audit Office (1992) suggest that some health authorities' manpower estimates and bids for Project 2000 funding may have been based on inappropriate staffing patterns, primarily due to the absence of an up to date comprehensive evaluation of the mix of staff required to meet the service needs. Furthermore, Elkan et al (1993) report how in some areas, a high proportion of registered nursing staff amongst replacement staff has resulted in reduced overall staffing levels due to the higher unit cost of the qualified nurse. The knock-on effect of this for standards of patient care is obvious (Elkan et al., 1993).

Leonard and Jowett (1990) report that the main areas for concern of service managers in the six demonstration sites studied were staffing level costs, skill mix, and the funding of support staff training. In particular, the assumption that replacement staff who would be permanent would be more efficient than students constantly rotating through placement areas was called into question. However, the assumption that the Project 2000 students would be less efficient than their traditional counterparts was borne out in practice (Jowett et al., 1994). The authors also report difficulties with the 20% service contribution allowed for in the Department's formula for replacing the pre-Project 2000 workforce, stating that this estimate was: "clearly not a reality in many cases" (p. 73). In this report, senior service and educational managers alleged that the whole structure on which these calculations were built subsequently became skewed by the whole gamut of changes that occurred as a result of the NHS reforms. Indeed, one ward sister claimed that the planned replacement programme had ground to a halt with the advent of Trust status (Jowett et al., 1994).

It would also appear that there are many inconsistencies in the costs of the actual link with higher education. The NAO (1992) point out that in some cases:

> ...colleges had decided to buy teaching and accommodation from their associated higher education institution in addition to meeting the basic charges relating to examination fees and library facilities (NAO, 1992, p. 31).

However, staff in a number of colleges visited by the NAO said that they were unclear about how to ensure they got maximum benefit from their associations with higher education, or what level of costs were appropriate. The costs of establishing and maintaining the higher education links were also an issue for nurse managers and educators in Jowett et al's (1994) study. These costs were reported to have been higher than expected and funding in this area was seen to be very much inadequate by the college principals interviewed. In particular, unforeseen travel costs and library costs were identified as being the most problematic (Jowett et al., 1994). In this regard, Bentley (1996), in a discussion of the official reports and documents preceding the implementation of Project 2000, directs criticism at their authors for failing to address "the subject of the increased costs involved in providing educational facilities needed to enable student nurses to achieve diploma level qualifications." (p. 134).

Student Funding on Project 2000

Project 2000 differs from the traditional programme in that it places greater emphasis on wider aspects of health such as health education, illness prevention and community care. It also changes the status of the student nurse (NAO, 1992). Traditional student nurses were health service employees and part of the nursing workforce and therefore paid a salary. Project 2000 students on the other hand are college based and are for the most part supernumerary to service. To emphasise their supernumerary standing and student status, remuneration is by way of a non-means tested training grant. This is also significant as traditional students by virtue of the fact that they were salaried, were therefore also connected to the negotiating machinery associated with staff pay. This is not the case for Project 2000 students. The education component of this grant, which was estimated to be 80% (Bentley, 1996), was to be paid to colleges by regions "once a contract for the number of students in a given year was agreed." (p.135). Burnard and Chapman (1990) give an example of a typical student bursary for those who commenced their programme in the original 13 English demonstration Project 2000 courses in the autumn of 1989. These are depicted in Table 1.3.

It was agreed that Project 2000 students receiving these bursaries were not to be liable for income tax, national insurance or superannuation contributions. However, they were expected to pay 20% of their personal community charge (poll tax) as is the case for all other students. Allowances were also made for those students with dependants, and current NHS staff who enter the Project 2000 programme were to retain their present salary rather than receive a bursary (Burnard and Chapman, 1990).

TABLE 1.3. Student bursaries in Project 2000 in the original demonstration districts

	London:	£4700
• Under 26 years at the start of the course—	Elsewhere:	£4000
	London:	£5200
• Age 26 and over at the start of the course—	Elsewhere:	£4500

Source: **Burnard and Chapman,** *Nurse Education: The Way Forward,* **1990.**

Problems with Student Funding

Despite the fact that these remuneration arrangements were perceived as being the most appropriate by both the statutory nursing bodies and by the Department of Health, a number of problems arose. Some difficulties arose in the manner in which the Project 2000 bursaries were managed particularly in situations where districts using the same college adopted different approaches. The National Audit Office (1992) cite the example of Shropshire and North Staffordshire College, where one district allowed the college to administer the students' bursaries while the other administered the bursaries themselves. The difficulty here is that problems can arise where districts allocate their own share of funds, especially if all parties cannot agree on priorities for funding.

It would also appear that there was some element of resentment on the part of some traditional students regarding the financial arrangements for Project 2000 students. For example, Elkan et al (1993) report how some Project 2000 students had a poor welcome from certain traditional students who, among other things, were envious of their education conditions. In particular the authors report how a few considered that Project 2000 students did not earn their bursary. There was also some resentment of the fact that the new students were required to pay only 20% of the poll tax. Traditional students, because they were salaried, were required to pay it in full. One student comment in this regard was:

> There's the argument (from traditional students) that we don't do any work for our pennies. I think initially it was that they thought that we were on a doss really. We come out with more than them at the end, a diploma, and we don't have to pay all the poll tax, yet they're doing a lot more actual physical work than us (Elkan et al, 1993, p. 60).

It must be emphasised however, that on the whole, Project 2000 students were in time welcomed and treated respectfully by both qualified staff and traditional students (Elkan et al, 1993; Jowett et al., 1994). Furthermore, it would appear that many of the friction's that did occur, happened early on in the programme and at a time when there was much ignorance regarding Project 2000 (Elkan et al, 1993). In particular, there were many fears that Project 2000 qualified nurses were going to be fast-tracked to all the lucrative jobs and hence, traditional students and existing qualified staff would be left behind and marginalised (Jowett et al., 1994). As will be seen later, this was not to be the case.

There are many other problems concerning student bursaries reported in the literature, not least the problem of student poverty. Indeed, it would appear that since bursaries were introduced in 1989, they have only been increased once (Willis, 1996). For example, a *No Limits* survey (Nursing Standard, 1996), suggests that nearly 80% of student nurses say that poverty is the greatest issue that affects them. Further, half of the respondents in this survey said that they would appreciate advice on where to get debt counselling in order to help them deal with financial concerns. When asked how the plight of today's

17

student nurse could be improved, almost one third said better accommodation while over 60% said they needed advice on how to maintain a healthy diet on such a small income. Of most concern was the finding that loneliness affected over one fifth of these students, while almost 50% felt they needed relationship counselling. The implications of these findings on student morale and on recruitment into the profession are also discussed in this report (Nursing Standard, 1996). In a similar survey carried out by the Nursing Times that same year, more money, affordable accommodation and better fringe benefits were among the issues raised by respondents. One such respondent, a second year student, said that:

> Subsidised accommodation has to be provided. In 1993 the Department of Health said that, strictly speaking, Project 2000 students did not need subsidised accommodation. But it's impossible here in north London. We live on £455 a month and even the cheapest accommodation is £60 a week before bills,...your left with nothing (Nursing Times, 1996,p. 31).

One of the goals of Project 2000 was to attract prospective students from non-traditional sources such as males, people from ethnic minorities, and older candidates (NAO, 1992; Jowett, 1994). This was primarily due to fears that a demographic timebomb, (namely the expectation that the numbers of suitably qualified female school leavers was about to fall drastically), was about to explode (Dolan, 1993). When one considers the increased likelihood that older candidates may have dependants such as spouses and/or children, it is unlikely that the above statement is going to serve as an attraction to them to enter nursing. Indeed, the RCN (1994) report that one third of nursing students are now over 25 years, and over 25% have dependent children.

There are also reports of problems in the funding of students on pre-registration degree programmes. These students, unlike Project 2000 students, do not receive a bursary. Rather they receive a much smaller means tested grant the same as a university student in any other discipline. An example of the type of financial problems this poses for students is given by Wells-Jansz, (1996). The author, a second year pre-registration degree student, claims that most undergraduate nursing students are forced to survive on a maximum grant of £1,820 per annum, that is if they qualify for it in the first place. Wells-Jansz goes on to compare the situation of a typical undergraduate nursing student and an undergraduate non-nursing student, pointing out that it costs a non-nursing undergraduate degree student £3,807 for an average year, while it costs an undergraduate nursing degree student between £4,511 and £5,412 per year. The main difference being the extra costs incurred by shoes, uniforms, travel to and from placements, and accommodation. The author argues that since the maximum grant available to these nursing students is £1,820, even with a full student loan (£1,385), most face a shortfall of about £2,000. The figure for non-nursing students is estimated to be £600. As a result, many nursing students either have to depend on their parents to help out financially, or else they have to take up evening and/or weekend jobs. The author cites a scenario described by a second year colleague:

> I don't sleep on Fridays,... I come to college for 9am and then go directly to work for the night shift at a local nursing home, till 8am on Saturday morning. I also work the night shift on Saturday and if possible a back shift on the Sunday, which finishes at 10pm and back to college for 9am on Monday (Wells-Jansz, 1996, p.52).

This issue of students needing to take on part-time work is also reported by Jowett et al's (1994) study of Project 2000 students, and by Willis' (1996) report of the RCNs Association of Nursing Students 1996 Annual Conference. Both these authors' reports concur with the assertion that unlike students from other disciplines, nurses do not have the benefit of long summer holidays in which to undertake work. Therefore, part-time employment has to be combined with their studies and practical placements (Sloper, 1994). Needless to say, studying full-time and working part-time causes great stress for students and is one of the common reasons why students consult the RCN's counselling service according to Snell, (1995).

Another difficulty encountered by pre-registration degree nurses is that they cannot claim any of the other benefits that are available to those on low income because they are on bursaries. This was well illustrated by one respondent in the Nursing Times study cited earlier, a third year pre-registration degree student and mother of three small children:

> Although my income is low enough to qualify for family credit, help with school dinners and free prescriptions, I cannot claim them as I am on a bursary. It's the fringe benefits of being on a low income that you lose when you are a student; the things that make life a bit more tolerable (Nursing Times, 1996,p. 31).

While it is true to say that much of the foregoing is anecdotal and is based on individual student's testimonies and hence its generalisability is questionable, the issue of student funding is one that has also been addressed at a national level by a number of eminent nurse leaders. For instance, Betty Kershaw, President of the Royal College of Nursing, in an open letter, urged Sir Ron Dearing of the Dearing Inquiry into higher education, to take seriously the concerns of all students over funding, adding that the particular circumstances of students of nursing should also be addressed (Kershaw, 1996). Similarly, Christine Hancock (1996), General Secretary of the RCN draws attention to the current situation whereby many newly qualified nurses, as well as having to negotiate their pay at a local level, also have to pay back the student loans they took out in order to financially support themselves through college.

This problem of student loans is one which has received a considerable amount of attention in the popular nursing press over the past year or so. Much of the concern stems from a Labour Party proposal in 1996 to transform what they term "the inadequate student loans system." (Willis, 1996). The government are proposing that students contribute to the financing of their education by paying back, through a progressive and income contingent system, probably through national insurance. While it would appear that the National Union of Students (NUS) favour these arrangements, there has been considerable resistance voiced by nursing unions and student bodies at the prospect of introducing these arrangements into nursing education (Willis, 1996). Willis goes on to cite a number of the concerns expressed by nursing bodies. For example, the author cites an RCN survey which reports that 65% of nursing students state that loans would affect their decision to enter higher education, while 24% say that they would avoid such loans at all costs, even if it meant not undertaking nurse training. The biggest concern is the expected difficulty of paying back these loans when one is not guaranteed a job after qualifying. Indeed, Hancock draws attention to the dilemma encountered by some nurses in trying to pay off such loans due to their inability to secure anything more than a short-term contract. The writer goes on to argue that this situation is unlikely to assist efforts to improve recruitment into the profession (Hancock, 1996). Willis (1996) does point out that while as of yet there has been no suggestion that the current bursary system will be affected, there is an argument that all nursing students should be funded in the same way, namely through a system of means-tested grants and top up loans, as is the current case for pre-registration degree students. It would appear that such a route is imminent due to the fact that most colleges are gradually moving towards full integration with higher education. Kershaw (1996) argues that all student nurses should have bursaries and not loans, suggesting that the Dearing Committee should consider them as a special case, as should students training for other vocational qualifications such as medicine, teaching and allied health professions, not least because they provide about 1000 hours service in their final year of training. However, the author emphasises the importance of nurse education remaining under the auspices of the Department of Health as she believes that this would help ensure that the practical side of the course would be accorded the same value as the academic part (Kershaw, 1996; cited in Willis, 1996).

1.5 Outcomes of Project 2000

Many hopes were vested in Project 2000 both in terms of what it would do for the professionalisation of nursing, and also in terms of it's outcomes for the health care needs of the British people in the new millennium. The goals set out for Project 2000 have already been discussed and can be seen to be wide ranging and radical. What is of crucial importance now for all concerned is, to what extent have these goals and dreams been realised? This is a vital question according to Naish (1993) and one that must be responded to with a "watertight" answer if nursing is to justify its costly new training programme. Alas, such answers are not readily forthcoming primarily due to the fact that there is as yet a paucity of research that explores the outcomes of Project 2000 or that demonstrates its impact on the type of nurse practitioner being produced (Casey, 1996; Fitzpatrick, et al., 1993). There is some evidence however, that at least some of the goals of Project 2000 are being attained, and clearly, it is too early yet to evaluate some of the expected outcomes of the programme, particularly those relating to the medium to long-term career paths of Project 2000 prepared nurses.

In 1992, shortly after the first cohort of Project 2000 prepared nurses qualified, the National Audit Office reported that while there were still some concerns that these nurses' practical skills may be deficient, early indications suggested that the new curriculum was making a positive impact on nursing practice (NAO, 1992). Similarly, Jasper, (1996) in a small study of eight staff nurses who had undergone Project 2000 education in one of the original demonstration districts, concluded that the UKCCs vision for the new curriculum was likely to be realised.

Jasper, using a phenomenological approach, found that these nurses:

> had gained the competent technical and clinical skills expected of any nurse....[and that] they also displayed skills previously absent in newly qualified nurses, such as evidence of analytical decision-making and confident interpersonal skills (Jasper, 1996, p. 779).

While the author asserts that the nurses were competent, she does point out that the process that they had experienced to attain this level of practice was at times traumatic. While the results help to illuminate the experiences of some of the first cohort of Project 2000 students, one must interpret them with some caution due to the small sample size, and also due to the self-report nature of the method used to collect the data.

Jowett et al., (1994) report that, when asked directly about their views on whether or not Project 2000 would create a different type of nurse, the majority of students felt that it would. Among the changes anticipated by the students, were an increase in confidence, depth of knowledge, adoption of a more holistic approach to care, less inclination to adhere to routines and, a more patient centred approach. Indeed, some of these attributes were prophesised for Project 2000 prepared nurses. For example, Allen (1993) suggested that the student centred learning approach adopted in the Project 2000 curriculum would lead to student empowerment which in turn would empower patients and lead to patient centred care. Similarly, Orr (1987) felt that the new programme would encourage students to embrace and build upon a body of knowledge that would ultimately inform practice. Indeed, Jowett et al., (1994) report that nurse educators felt that the Project 2000 students had a greater depth and breath of knowledge compared with traditionally educated nurses. These teachers also reported that the students were highly motivated, thinking critically, analytically and reflectively about nursing practice, and had highly developed academic skills. Likewise, Hickey (1996) in his study of traditionally trained nurses' perceptions of Project 2000, found that some respondents (albeit a minority), felt that the course would produce nurses with improved academic and research skills.

Other changes anticipated by students in Jowett et al's (1994) study were that they would be kinder and more respectful to patients, and would want to change nursing practice. In this latter regard, one respondent feared that they might end up "banging their heads against a brick wall" as a result of their efforts to change things (p.103). Indeed, many of the nurse teachers interviewed by Payne et al., (1991) feared that this would be the case suggesting that in time Project 2000 nurses could become socialised into maintaining the status quo and that the Project 2000 promise to nursing might not be realised. Recent evidence corroborates this fear, with an ENB survey reporting that 49% of the newly qualified practitioners stated that they were unable to influence practice (ENB, 1996). Regarding the expectation that nurses would nurse more sensitively, Slevin (1995) in a comparative study of the attitudes of traditionally trained nurses and Project 2000 nurses towards people with learning disabilities, found that Project 2000 nurses who had had a placements with these clients, demonstrated more positive attitudes towards them.

Notwithstanding the above, there is also some evidence that Project 2000 nurses did in fact have some deficiencies in clinical practice. Elkan et al (1993) in discussing the Department's replacement formula, question whether Project 2000 students enhance practice in a similar way to traditional students, arguing that the evidence suggests that Project 2000 students are acquiring confidence and competence in clinical practice at a much later stage in their training than traditional students. The authors point out that:

> Whereas traditional students, by their second year, were judged by many service staff to be capable of making a significant and valuable contribution to the work of the ward team, Project 2000 students in the fourth term of their Common Foundation Programme (CFP) are still seen very much as novices and their contribution deemed much more limited at that stage than that of traditional students. Until they undertake their final rostered' stage of their training, Project 2000 students simply do not have the same exposure to the practical ward setting as traditional students (Elkan et al., 1993, p. 22).

Many other writers concur with this position, most notably Elzubier and Sherman, (1995) and Elkan et al., (1993). These latter authors quote one students comments regarding the fear of practice that this lack of confidence has generated:

We're worried about our practical skills. When we get on the ward we'll be expected to do the same as a staff nurse. And I'm worried that we're not going to be able to do as much as they do. Because they've had three years practical training. I mean everybody says "Oh, you'll catch up very quickly on your practical training", but I mean I know I'm going to be anxious when I get onto a ward.... (Elkan et al., 1993, p. 63).

While similar fears were expressed by students in Jowett et al's (1994) study, the authors report how only a handful of nurse teachers considered students' competence and confidence in practice to be an area of concern, and also, a majority of the students later commented that when they qualified, they no longer had any real doubts about coping with their responsibilities as a staff nurse.

Furthermore, even in the rostered period at the end of year three, Project 2000 students were deemed to be in need of more supervision and guidance than their traditional third year counterparts. It was generally felt that they could not be relied upon at least for the first part of this period (Jowett et al., 1994). The authors also report that in some cases wards would book extra staff if Project 2000 students were on rostered placements.

While there is little evidence by which to judge these students' quality of practice, on the whole however, the students have expressed satisfaction with at least some aspects of the course. Jasper (1996) reports that, while there were some reservations about certain organisational issues, students were very satisfied with the value, breath and relevance of the course. Likewise, Jowett et al., (1994) report that all of the students interviewed were able to identify positive gains from the course, particularly with regard to self confidence and self-awareness. Indeed at their end of the three year study, the authors also report how all of the staff concerned, also presented a very positive image of their encounters with Project 2000 students, and of their hopes and expectations for the future success of the programme. Perhaps the best yardstick by which to measure the students evaluation of the course is the degree to which they would recommend the course to others. Indeed, Jowett et al., (1994) found that most students interviewed would recommend the course to a friend, however that it was not to be undertaken lightly. The students concluded that the course could prove to be extremely rewarding if approached in a realistic manner.

1.6   Transition to Work

There is a dearth of literature on the experiences of newly qualified Project 2000 nurses' transition to practice, however, one such study (Jasper, 1996), albeit one with a small sample (n=8), is useful in assisting one to understand the experiences of such a group of nurses, and hence is used to structure the discussion here. Jasper (1996), using a qualitative approach that was informed by phenomenological methodology, studied the experiences of a group of eight staff nurses who had been students in the first cohort of a Project 2000 course in one of the original demonstration districts. The researcher, using taped focused group discussions and semi-structured interviews, identified six themes from the data analysed:

Theme One-Coming Out of School

Here, the differences between nursing as a student and as a qualified nurse are described in terms of how well prepared nurses felt for their new role. All respondents drew attention to the discrepancy between what they were told to expect of their abilities on qualifying, and what they found upon qualification. Qualification was experienced as a complete role change and not just as a transition, as was expected. There was very much a feeling of being thrown in at the deep end, however, soon after qualifying, there appeared to be a realisation that they had a deep knowledge base, and this gave way to a more favourable appraisal of their own competence as a staff nurse in that they perceived themselves to be functioning effectively in the new role. Jasper draws attention to the fact that this feeling of lack of preparedness for the staff nurse role is not peculiar to Project 2000 nurses, citing a number of studies that demonstrate this finding from other research contexts (Rundell, 1990; Lathlean, 1987; Walker, 1986; Gott, 1984, and Simpson, 1979). The author draws attention to the finding however, that unlike subjects in other studies, Project 2000 graduates do not appear to be lacking in skills such as decision making, the ability to challenge others confidently, and analytical thinking (Jasper, 1996).

Theme Two-Living in the Real World

In this theme, the overwhelming impression was that the nurses were disappointed with reality as they found it. The reality of the staff nurse role contrasted greatly with their pre-qualifying impression, in particular in regard to their inability to deliver care to the standard that they would wish. This lead to frustration and demoralisation, and seven of the eight nurses suggested that they became resigned to the situation, having decided to stop confronting the system in the interests of their own survival (Jasper, 1996). Elkan and Robinson (1993) warned of this risk of the theory-practice gap confounding the success of Project 2000 due to its maintenance of routineised care. This type of reality shock has also been the experience of graduate nurses from degree programmes (Sinclair, 1987 and Luker, 1984), and like these Project 2000 students, graduate nurses were also observed to manipulate their environment in order to survive (Luker, 1984). This, according to Jasper (1996) appears to have lead to an increase in faith in ones judgement, to an ability to confront others within the workplace, and to the maintenance of a perspective under pressure with the simultaneous development of interpersonal skills to achieve these.

Theme Three — the Effect of the Label

This theme came about as a result of the impression given by the nurses that the label of "Project 2000" was like a millstone around their necks. These were among the first to qualify as nurses through the Project 2000 route and not surprisingly therefore, were the focus of much attention. One respondent in Jaspers (1996) study commented:

> I felt a little pressure being the first Project 2000 [student] here- you felt the eyes on your back
> as if someone is watching you- whether that is true in hindsight... (Jasper, 1996, p. 785).

Indeed there is much evidence that many of the Project 2000 educated nurses received a hostile reception from traditionally prepared staff and students (Jowett et al., 1994; Clegg, 1992; Dolan, 1991; Casey, 1990 and Naish, 1990). It would appear that the chief reason for this was fear of the unknown, and lack of preparation of these staff for Project 2000 nurses. There was also the belief, cited by Luker (1984), that traditionally prepared nurses held that there is an inverse relationship between academic endowment and the ability to participate in hands on nursing care. The author continues:

> Whilst the belief has no factual foundation, it is perpetuated through the apprenticeship system
> where pursuit of knowledge is secondary to practical experience (Luker, 1984, p. 6-7).

23

This view was one that was also reported as being "widely held" among service staff and traditionally trained students in Elkan et al's., (1993) study. There was concern that Project 2000 nurses, while possessing a sophisticated theoretical understanding of nursing, would have little practical competence by which to deliver actual nursing care. Clearly, this attitude rubbed off on the nurses as evidenced by such comments as:

> There is a derogatory attitude towards us. ....that we know it all; that we can't do anything; that we just stand around; that we know all the theory but can't even empty a bedpan, that sort of stuff.

and:

> There's like a stigma against us. Like yesterday we went to get our off-duty for our next placements. And we said 'we're student nurses' and of course they looked down the RGN list and said 'Oh, I can't see your names.' So we had to say 'We're Project 2000 students.' .... (Elkan et al., 1993, p. 60-1).

In time however, it would appear that the nurses were able to rationalise these comments as being directed at the label rather that at them in person (Jasper, 1996). Also, despite the fact that all of the respondents in the Jowett et al., study were able to recall events in which hostility had been directed at them, most said that this abated over time, as service staff and traditional students got to know more about Project 2000 and to see the students in the practice setting. However, Jasper (1996) reports that the constant pressure did take its toll, particularly in terms of its attack on nurses confidence. Moreover, it would appear that much of this hostility could have been prevented if adequate preparation of traditional staff had been provided at the outset.

Evidence was also given of positive attitudes being expressed towards these nurses especially in regard to their ability to practice competently, and these Jasper reports served well in boosting confidence. Some comments in this regard from the Elkan et al., (1993) study were:

> The (traditional) students on the ward I did my placement on were really good. It was always the (traditional) students on the ward that I was on that would take me round and show me how to do things.

and:

> The sister and the (traditional) student nurses on ward x were absolutely brilliant. They were my support, along with a couple of the staff nurses. The third year students on the ward were the support of everything (Elkan et al., 1993, p. 61).

Jasper (1996) lays much of the blame for this situation of negative labelling, on the hurried implementation of Project 2000. This labelling arose chiefly as a result of there not being enough time in many cases, for service staff to be adequately prepared for receiving Project 2000 nurses, nor for them to express their fears and concerns regarding the implications of Project 2000 for their qualifications and promotability. Studies of graduate nurse preparation also bear testimony to such labelling (Sinclair, 1987 and Luker, 1984). Fortunately, Jasper (1996) reports, the strategies employed by these nurses for managing such reactions towards them have lead to an ability on their part to function effectively in whatever environment they find themselves working. It has lead to the development of a sophisticated repertoire of interpersonal skills, the author contends. Jasper continues:

> It appears that the educational philosophy of the course has become deep rooted, and that the nurses have the capacity to fulfil the expectations of the UKCC(1986) in terms of flexibility in practice, and have the capacity to give, as well as supervise, nursing care. (Jasper, 1996, p.785).

Theme Four — Learning to Cope

In this theme, the development of the nurses coping strategies is charted, particularly in regard to the management of people and patient care. Jasper (1996) details how the inaugural response of nurses to their new role was one of terror, and how this gradually subsided and the nurses soon eased into their new roles. Once accepted however, evidence is that nurses looked on the role in an extremely serious way, "as if the nurses were aware of the trust placed in them as a result of qualification, which they were determined not to abuse" (p. 786). Similarly, Jowett et al., (1994) found that the majority of respondents in their study also felt able to cope with their staff nurse role. Overall, about one third of the nurses felt that their transition to work had been uneventful, and the other two thirds, while admitting to some initial insecurities and concerns, felt that these gradually diminished. Like their counterparts in Jasper's study, their concerns were mainly to do with the prospect of being placed in charge of the ward, and with being held accountable for care given. One respondent in Jowett et al's., study commented:

> I wasn't confident at all and I did find it really difficult to adjust and it was very difficult to break the habit of knowing that there was someone to help you and that you didn't have to do everything perfectly because it wasn't your responsibility and suddenly you qualify and you are out on your own [sic] (Jowett et al., 1994, p. 99).

Jasper (1996) goes on to point out how much of the nurses ability to cope came about as a result of their development of the skills necessary to challenge and to manipulate situations they encountered in practice. She continues to suggest that the result of these abilities were evident in the substantial amount of change that they had managed to bring about despite being at an early stage of career development.

Jasper comments:

> Although it appears that the nurses have the knowledge and skills to attempt to change practice, they have to use the tactics and strategies of challenge and manipulation....rather than use direct suggestions which could be seen as openly contradicting authority figures (Jasper, 1996, p. 786).

Jasper (1996) argues that this theme is important as it indicates the nurses ability to extend their practice from that of care delivery, to the management of people and patients, and also, the ability to contest, and be influential and innovative in their work. Indeed, Jowett et al, (1994) report that many of the Project 2000 students that they interviewed said that they wanted to bring about changes in nursing practice. However, at least one of these students anticipated that she might find herself banging her head against a brick wall in attempting to do so. Similarly, many of the nurse teachers that were interviewed by Payne et al., (1991) feared that this in fact would prove to be the case, resulting in a situation whereby within a short space of time, these nurses would be forced to conform to the status quo of ritualistic nursing care.

Perhaps some measure of the nurses ability to manage and deliver patient care is however, that both authors report that the majority of the nurses were given varying degrees of responsibility from an early stage with apparently successful outcomes (Jasper, 1996; Jowett et al., 1994).

Theme Five — Us and Them

This theme illustrates the perception among the Project 2000 nurses that they were different from nurses trained through other routes, while at the same time emphasising their desire to be the same as well as different from them. The desire "to be the same" stems from the wish to be able to execute their role as competently as other staff nurses do, while the emphasis on difference comes about from the belief that they possess abilities over and above the other nurses. One respondents comment in this regard was: "Hopefully I felt that I had a stronger theoretical foundation to build on, however, initially the idea was to get out there and work as a staff nurse." (Jasper, 1996, p. 786). These nurses had developed a different set of attitudes particularly in regard to a more holistic approach to care, and a more favourable disposition towards the need for a sound theoretical base for practice. Such attitudes frequently clashed with those operant in the clinical area, and the Project 2000 nurses suggested that they often found themselves caught in the middle of the inconsistent beliefs and values held by clinical and teaching staff. The nurses also looked upon their new higher qualification as an entity in and of itself, and one that accorded them significant benefits over and above the benefits one might expect with a traditional nurse qualification (Jasper, 1996). It has been suggested however, that when new graduates experience such a hostile environment at work, "fitting in" might require them to downplay the content of their education. As Fitzpatrick and colleagues put it:

> It would thus appear that a dichotomy exists whereby students of nursing exposed to a broader experience and an improved knowledge base rooted in sound research are inhibited in their application of this knowledge and skill in the practice setting (Fitzpatrick, While and Roberts, 1993, p. 1491).

The authors concluded however, that when the nurse graduate population increases, opinion towards this group may become more favourable. While Project 2000 qualified nurses are not graduates in the strict sense of the word, it is likely that such an opinion change towards them may also occur in time.

Jasper (1996) asserts the findings of her small study demonstrates that Project 2000 nurses are capable of both giving and supervising nursing care, and that the course has produced a nurse who is capable of standing firmly as an equal member of the mulitdisciplinary team. The author concludes that nurses educated in this way will retain and exercise their preferred philosophy of care once in practice. It would appear however, that if a greater effort had been made to prepare service staff for Project 2000, and also, if a period of preceptored practice had been provided for, much of the trauma outlined above, might not have occurred. Indeed, this latter issue was one that was given much consideration after the first cohorts of Project 2000 qualified. Included in the UKCCs initial proposals for Project 2000 was a recommendation that the Council proceed to review post-registration nursing education and practice. In November, 1991, when this review was complete, as well as announcing the proposals, the Council recommended that all newly qualified nurses, both traditional and Project 2000, should receive a four month period of support from a preceptor after registration, in order to assist with the transition from student to practitioner (NAO, 1992). In July the following year, the Department of Health announced its support for these proposals, and according to the NAO; " From April 1993 all National Health Service employers will be *encouraged* to provide preceptors for new practitioners..." (NAO, 1992, p. 26-7. [my italics]). Elkan et al., (1993) suggest that such proposals are a natural progression from Project 2000 proposals, however, their interpretation was that a period of six months was being advocated by the Council. In any case, it would appear that not all Project 2000 nurses had a preceptor available to them when they first qualified. For instance, Jowett et al., (1994) report that up to three-fifths of respondents in their final evaluation study were not appointed a preceptor, while another fifth "could not identify any impact of their (preceptors') functioning..... had seen no evidence of it.," (p. 100), this despite the fact that these nurses had been told that such a system was in place. The final fifth did however have a positive experience of their preceptorship arrangements and it would also appear that others, while not necessarily having been allocated a preceptor, were given some form of induction, and did report that they found senior ward staff helpful in terms of aiding their transition to work.

Of some concern however, is the suggestion that some personnel, both students, qualified staff and non-nursing staff, appear to have interpreted these preceptor proposals as confirmation of the view that Project 2000 students on graduation, are not yet competent to take on the full responsibilities of a staff nurse (Elkan et al., 1993). The fear here is that if health authorities cannot be guaranteed competence, they may instead employ other workers such as health care assistants, instead of newly qualified nursing personnel, as they know that these personnel are coming with clear competencies in that they are trained to NVQ level.

1.7 The Changing Role of Nurse Educators

The implementation of Project 2000 had enormous implications for all concerned, not least for nurse teachers. Clearly, some nurse teachers thrived during the change process, however, it would also appear that many struggled to keep up with the pace of change, and indeed, some succumbed (Jowett et al., 1994). A comment by Robinson (1993), based on the author's own research findings, illuminates some of the variables associated with this great change, and how it affected nurse teachers:

> For many nurse teachers, even those who welcomed Project 2000 with positive optimism, the reality of its early implementation,...meant a working world turned upside-down with little direction and considerable confusion. There was a consequent loss of meaning to working roles, loss of stability and a diminishing sense of personal value (Robinson, 1993, p. 41).

The author argues that this situation was inevitable, given the magnitude of the changes associated with Project 2000, and also given the plethora of other changes associated with the health service reforms that were operant at the time. Nurse teachers in this study made frequent comment about feelings of loss of personal control such as "I feel totally out of control of the situation", "too many variables to control," "being deskilled," and so on, giving some appreciation of the stress that many of them felt, especially during the initial implementation period.

In this section, some of the stresses associated with these major changes will be analysed, as will some of the positive aspects of the change that were also evident from the literature on the role and role changes encountered by nurse teachers.

Calls for Graduate Status

One of the greater sources of stress was the implications for nurse teachers of the proposal by the UKCC in 1986 and adopted by the ENB in 1989, that all nurse teachers would be required to hold at least a first degree. The rationale for this was that if nursing schools were going to be linked to higher education and in part validated by them, and also, if courses were to be upgraded to diploma level, then nurse teachers would have to hold an academic qualification at least one level higher than that at which they were teaching (Charlwood, 1993). In order to meet this demand for graduate status, a number of degree courses were planned and developed which were particularly aimed at nurse teachers (Carlisle, 1991).

With regard to what type of degree was deemed best for nurse teachers, opinions varied. The UKCC (1987), in calling for graduate status for nurse teachers, suggest that this need not necessarily be in teaching, however, Scott-Wright et al.,(1979) emphasise that these degrees should be in nursing, and preferably at a post graduate level. These latter authors argue that teachers should be experts in the subject matter that they teach. Similarly, it is suggested that nurse teachers should have a primary degree in nursing, with a specialist qualification in an area related to one of the Project 2000 branch programmes (Nurse Education Today, 1987). In this editorial, the writer goes on to suggest that a teacher training course, in addition to the prospective nurse teacher's professional and academic qualifications, is not feasible and is also unnecessary due to the fact that all nurses should have some preparation in practical teaching skills. However, the author does concede that some nurse teachers may choose to specialise in education and that these teachers' contribution will continue to be essential.

While it is unclear just how many nurse teachers were graduates at the outset of Project 2000, Payne et al., (1991) report that over 25% of the nurse teachers interviewed at an early stage in their research had a first and/or a higher degree, and more than one third were currently studying for a first or higher degree, with many more planning to embark on such studies in the near future. Many of these nurse teachers were funding themselves in the absence of a contribution from their employer, or in cases where funding was too slow to materialise (Payne et al., 1991). Clearly, teachers considered that there was indeed an urgency for them to become graduates. This sense of urgency according to Payne et al., (1991), not alone came from the ENB (1989) proposal, but also from the perception that nurse teachers needed to be seen as having academic credibility in the eyes of their higher education counterparts. Indeed, this perception was well founded as there have been suggestions that staff in higher education did in fact question the qualifications of the nurse teachers in terms of their ability to teach in higher education (Jowett et al., 1994). Moreover, the Royal College of Nursing's Commission on Nursing Education (1985), which also called for graduate status for nurse teachers, commented that colleges of nurse education would not normally procure accreditation for its diploma course unless or until the majority of the relevant teachers attained graduate status. Furthermore, whilst accepting the need for nurse teachers to become graduates, Owen (1988), argues that nurse academics who hold degrees have much to offer higher education in that they have the combined advantages of nursing and academic qualifications and often a much wider range of experience that other academics. The author asserts that they are therefore more than capable of taking the academic lead in their area in creating and teaching new courses.

The urgency to attain degrees was not without its problems. Payne et al., (1991) report how some staff felt that too many nurse teachers were attending college at once with the result that there were not enough left behind to do the work. This lead to a situation whereby the work of the colleges of nursing was slowed down, this at a time when the pace of developments was rapid. There are also reports of staff becoming over stressed due to the pressure they felt in attaining graduate status (Jowett et al., 1994, Charlwood, 1993), and this is not surprising given the nature and context of all of these changes. This latter author commented:

> For many teachers, the need to achieve graduate status has simply added to the high levels of anxiety they were already experiencing at this time of change. Some have obtained degrees because they were under pressure to do so, rather than to achieve any personal ambition (Charlwood, 1993, p. 48).

Moreover, the author adds that many nurse teachers had to pursue a part-time degree as well as hold down a full-time job, this at a time when there was a substantial increase in workload as a result of involvement in the implementation of Project 2000. This factor also meant that they were precluded from experiencing university life resulting in them being in the odious position of wishing to impart the mores of higher education to their students without having being given the chance to experience these for themselves (Charlwood, 1993). Professional survival and the perception by many nurse teachers that it would be difficult for them to get a degree was, according to Gibbs and Rush (1987), also a contributory factor in the genesis of stress among nurse teachers. Jowett et al., (1994) reported how some nurse teachers were becoming particularly stressed due to the dual pressures of being expected to study for a degree (which had to be achieved by 1995), while at the same time being expected to participate in research as part requirement of their higher education role.

A Change in Teaching Focus

The Curriculum Revolution literature is extremely critical of the pedagogical teaching practices that are widespread in many areas of education including nursing (Allen, 1990a; Allen, 1990b; Bevis and Murray, 1990 and Diekelmann, 1990). According to Darbyshire, et al., (1990), the traditional "factory model" of nurse training, while producing nurses who supposedly could be relied upon to get the work done, did little for the profession of nursing, or for the personal and professional development of the individual student. Consequently, an androgogical approach was advocated by the planners of Project 2000 (UKCC, 1986). Andragogy, the theory and practice of educating adults, suggests that educators of adults must take account of the adult's wealth of personal experience, must make the subject matter clearly relevant to their needs, and must actively engage the adult learner in the learning process (Knowles, 1980). Perhaps the most important aspect of andragogy that is emphasised in the Project 2000 curriculum is that of student centred learning, and the allied concept of self directed learning. Student centred learning according to Burnard (1986) is closely associated with patient centred care. If the profession really believes in a process of nursing that enables people to regain their independence, then it is vitally important that nursing education allows students to retain their integrity as adults. Such approaches to learning represent a major paradigm shift, one according to Allen (1993), that represents a shift of perspective of stunning dimensions: "...an ideological shift in the way educators perceive students, in the way students perceive themselves, and eventually in the way that the nursing profession will see nursing and the role of the nurse." (Allen, 1993, p.58).

However, a number of researchers have discovered that not all learners are willing and/or able to take responsibility for their own learning (Burnard and Morrison, 1992; Vaughan, 1990 and Horsburgh, et al., 1989). Burnard and Morrison (1992) for example, found that students preferred more teacher direction and management of learning experiences, while teachers believed that students should take more responsibility for their own learning. This the authors argue, is because students have been socialised in their earlier educational experiences towards pedagogical approaches to teaching. The challenges to nurse teachers therefore, is to re-socialise their students towards student-centred learning methods, something that requires considerable resource and time investment on the part of the teacher. This is not always easy to achieve, and Elkan et al., (1993) report how the size of Project 2000 student intakes and the physical lack of enough rooms in which to teach them has sometimes thwarted attempts to use the small group teaching methods and other student centred approaches which both students and nurse teachers said they preferred.

Such a lack of resources have also been alluded to by other writers, notably, Payne and colleagues who commented that:

> ...intakes for Project 2000 were so large as to militate against what were seen as the best teaching methods [experiential learning, small-group work and role-play], and teachers had to resort to talk and chalk' because of the sheer weight of numbers (Payne et al., 1991, p. 4).

This situation, the authors report, portrayed a retrograde step for nurse education in the minds of many nurse teachers who had been using these methods with much success, prior to the implementation of Project 2000. Furthermore, it is a problem that was anticipated in advance of Project 2000 (Burnard and Chapman, 1990).

It is also evident however, that not all Project 2000 nurse teachers were willing to embrace the principles of the new curriculum (Crotty, 1993; Crotty and Butterworth, 1992 and Robinson, 1991) and Mason, (1991b) doubts whether in fact it is realistic to expect such principles to be incorporated by nurse teachers who themselves are products of a more traditional education system. Moreover, Darbyshire (1991) suggests that if these principles are to be operationalised in the new curriculum, the current method of nurse teacher preparation needs to be radically overhauled.

Student centred learning makes great demands on the teacher according to Prew (1989), such as the need to create a closer teacher-student relationship in which the teacher acknowledges and fosters each students learning needs. Elkan et al., (1993) report such a relationship at least from some of the Project 2000 students interviewed. Despite students initial reservations about their obligations in regard to self-directed learning, they acknowledged that the tutors had put a great deal of effort into supporting them in their studies. One student commented regarding such support:

> The thing that we have got here is so much tutor back-up. And they are so keen for it [Project 2000] to work. The tutors are absolutely excellent. ...If you are totally honest with them, there's a lot of support there. ... they will go out of their way, literally, to help you, and I don't think you could ask for more than that (Elkan et al., 1993, p. 55).

The authors also point out how other students, mainly those who seemed unable to take responsibility for their own learning, were not so fulsome in their praise of tutors.

Indeed many of these students complained of their tutors lack of support and direction. Moreover, the authors reported that while most tutors did their utmost to support those students who requested support, they were unable to offer long-term individual support to every student. As a result, many students, particularly those who were "least able to understand and put into practice 'self-directed learning,' "(p.56) floundered in their attempts to do so. The authors conclude that it was not the tutors inability to foster such principles that lead to a failure to give students guidance and goals towards which to aim, rather it was because they were overstretched and overworked (Elkan et al., 1993).

Increase in Workload

This issue of being overworked, particularly during the initial implementation period, is one that has emerged in a number of studies (Jowett et al., 1994; Elkan et al., 1993 and Payne et al., 1991). Payne et al., (1991) report how nurse teachers found the pace of change "ridiculous", somewhat analogous to "laying the lines while the train is coming" (p. 1). Most nurse teachers were still involved in running and teaching other programmes and hence found themselves exhausted with work when curriculum planning started in earnest. On top of this, many were also reading for first or higher degrees as discussed earlier. Elkan et al., (1993) report that many nurse teachers were working very long hours, and there is evidence from this study that as a result, their work was suffering. The authors point out that due to their workload, some teachers were unable to provide adequate tutor support, particularly in regard to their role as facilitators of self-directed learning. Moreover, with regard to the personal tutor role, Jowett et al., (1994) reported that many nurse teachers had between 6 and 20 students (although two had 28 and 48 respectively), and that such a level of student supervision put increasing pressure on nurse tutors, not to mention what it did for the quality of the support given. In addition, nurse teachers in Payne et al's., (1991) study expressed concerns that traditional students were being neglected as a result of nurse teachers having to absorb themselves in the new curriculum. The authors also state that another result of this work pressure was that the Project 2000 course structure and teaching was still being planned long after the common foundation programme had commenced, causing one senior nurse teacher to comment: "my chin is just lapping against the waterline" (p. 1). Nurse teachers also expressed concerns that this situation meant that there was no chance to iron out inconsistencies in the curriculum or in timetables until the course was underway.

Jowett et al., (1994) indicate how some nurse teachers found that the need to constantly update themselves in specialist areas, primarily due to the fact that they were now having to prepare and teach their subjects from a different perspective, placed "very great demands" on them (p.122). The authors suggest however, that this may have occurred as a result of the traditional philosophy in nurse education that the teacher should always know more than, and be ahead of their students, a philosophy they hasten to say, that is very much incongruous with that of the new course. In particular, nurse teachers were having to reorient their teaching towards a health based model (Gough, et al., 1993), as well as towards more adult centred approaches as discussed above. Indeed, Allen (1993), reports how students complained about how the health emphasis is managed by nurse teachers in a number of colleges. That some nurse teachers were also expected to participate in research as part of their role within higher education has been discussed earlier, and this also was a source of stress in terms of these teachers' workloads. Finally, it would also appear that teachers' personal lives suffered. Payne et al., (1991) describe how nurse teachers regularly worked late evenings and weekends, and did not take annual leave entitlements. Many respondents suggested that sick leave among nurse teachers had risen as a result of this pressure.

The Lack of Preparation

Allied to this increase in workload associated with Project 2000 is the lack of preparation that many nurse teachers felt during the initial implementation of the new curriculum. The consequences of the hasty start to the implementation of Project 2000 were frequently raised by nurse teachers in a number of studies (Jowett et al., 1994; Elkan et al, 1993 and Payne et al., 1991), and some of the implications of this rushed start have been or will be alluded to in this discourse. While there is some evidence that nurse teachers in a few areas were briefed on Project 2000 (Payne et al., 1991), the authors report that the majority of teachers interviewed said that they felt unprepared and unsure of their roles within the new curriculum. Also, it would appear that Project 2000 briefing sessions were few and far between and while many felt that they were *au fait* with the principles of the new programme, they were given no idea of the complexities involved in the changes (Payne et al., 1991). One commented that teaching staff were informed when in fact they should have been educated. Of interest was the feeling expressed by nurse teachers who held degrees and/or teaching qualifications. They felt that these experiences had served them well through the change process. Robinson (1993) reports that what teachers felt they required most throughout the process was more time, not just for preparation, but also to reflect on and acclimatise to the new demands placed upon them as a result of the new programme. They needed this time the author says, to help them to re-establish a sense of meaning, and this was summed up in one such teacher's comment: "The speed of implementation of the curriculum has produced an unstable monster; an enormous alien thing." (Robinson, 1993, p.43). Other teachers in this study requested that they be given time out to abreact and to reflect on what was happening, in order to enable them to prepare for what was yet to come. Moreover, Jowett et al., (1994) recounts that the "cut corners" and the "limited co-operative working" with the link institutions meant that those delivering the course were quite concerned about the quality of the provision, at least in the early stages. Furthermore in this regard, Jowett et al., (1994) point out how some staff confessed that the urgency had been so much that they had been unable to make a proper job of planning the curriculum and in particular that there was no time to be creative or reflective in their thinking. The authors further comment how the curriculum planning had been arbitrary with "people falling into roles by default" (p.58). One children's nurse teacher recounted how she was not consulted or involved in any way with the planning of the children's section of the Common Foundation Programme, while other teachers found themselves having to teach on courses to which they contributed nothing in the planning phase. Conversely, there were others who were not asked to teach on courses that they planned. Moreover, other teachers complained that work that they had contributed to the curriculum never materialised, or was changed without their consultation (Jowett et al., 1994).

While many nurse teachers appeared to lay much of the blame for this rushed start at the feet of management, it would appear that they too were given very little time in which to plan. The National Audit Office (1992) report that some of the organisations that they consulted, as well as many managers and staff in the health authorities and colleges that were visited, suggested that it would have been helpful to have had more notice of the commencement of Project 2000. Apparently, some sites were given less than six months notice. The result of this uncertainty was that strategic planning for both education and service was rushed and hence suffered. On recounting this finding to the Department of Health, the NAO were told that the government had to balance the needs of Project 2000 with those of the NHS as a whole (NAO, 1992).

The Need to Develop Clinical Credibility

In the UKCCs original Project 2000 document (UKCC, 1986), it is suggested that responsibility for teaching Project 2000 students in the clinical areas should not be left entirely to service staff. Rather, the Council envisaged that nurse teachers would also perform a clinical teaching role, however, Elkan et al., (1993) argue that the document is both brief and vague on this point. What the document says is that:

> Those staff who are employed as teachers must...possess an up-to-date overview and understanding of the care settings to which students are allocated and of the learning opportunities offered within them. This is essential if they are to serve as role models for students..... (UKCC, 1986, Para 7.29).

Additionally, Elkan et al., (1993) accuse the Council of neglecting to offer any advice on how nurse teachers might retain the knowledge and skills necessary to serve as such role models. The authors argue that while the Council appears to be suggesting that some kind of lecturer/practitioner role be developed, they are rather vague on the issue. This criticism is one that is echoed by Kirk, et al., (1997) who argue that clinical credibility needs to be clearly defined, and educational institutions need to place more emphasis on teachers' clinical development if the rhetoric of policy is to become a reality. It would also appear that colleges had failed to make adequate allowances in workload for nurse teachers' clinical role, yet have made available many study days for academic studies (Burke, 1993; Acton, et al., 1992). This the authors argue accentuates the worth of academic credibility over clinical credibility.

There appears to be little consensus on the part of nurse teachers regarding their role, if any, in clinical teaching. Jowett et al., (1994) report that nurse teachers were divided on the issue. They cite a comment by one nurse teacher respondent in their study that she was "not a clinician now but an educationalist" (p. 62) and that credibility could not be achieved or maintained without sustained and regular clinical contact. The authors further report how other nurse teachers suggested that they were first and foremost nurses and hence, nurse teachers must maintain a hands-on commitment. Towards the end of their study, Jowett et al., (1994) report that more and more nurse teachers had no ambition for a hands-on role since they did not see this as mandatory for nurse teaching. In some cases, especially in mental health and mental handicap, nurse teachers also felt that such a role was inappropriate and that they could add little to practical teaching, which they felt was best accomplished by expert clinical staff. Jones (1985) found that nurse teachers placed their clinical role low on the list of priorities in comparison to other aspects of their role. However, the author reports that they experienced considerable conflict and frustration over lack of time to develop this role. Similarly, Kirk et al., (1997), identified lack of time as the most frequently cited difficulty when it came to maintaining clinical expertise. However, unlike those in Jones' study, these latter teachers indicated that spending periods in the clinical environment updating their clinical skills, was "highly desirable" (p.1042). However, they did acknowledge that this was unlikely to happen. Kirk and colleagues further argue that, if pre-Project 2000 teachers found it difficult to maintain clinical credibility, it is unlikely that today's nurse teachers will be able to do so either, primarily due to their increased workload (Kirk et al., 1997). Indeed there is evidence that the increased workload of today's nurse teacher has in fact further reduced their clinical role (Clifford, 1992 and Robinson, 1991). This is also evident from Payne et al's., (1991) report whereby the authors recount how nurse teachers interviewed in their study, some of whom were described as "overwhelmed" by their other commitments, maintained a precarious balancing act in order to juggle the many demands on their clinical time. Most of the teachers in this study said that they could only spend a maximum of about half a day per week in their given clinical area, and much of this time was spent giving support and advice to clinical staff, and informing them on aspects of the course. They also alluded to feelings of frustration at having to stretch themselves so thinly. Indeed, some nurse teachers had to cease their clinical involvement due to other work pressures. Similarly, students who were interviewed in this study also indicated the lack of visibility of teachers in the clinical areas suggesting that those few visits that they did have, had little or no impact on clinical learning experience (Payne et al., 1991). Jowett et al., report how some junior nurse teachers were expected to spend as much as 20% of their time in the clinical areas, however, in reality, this was rarely achieved. These teachers felt that other demands on their time meant that their efforts in the clinical areas was insufficient to enable them to attain clinical credibility, or even, to enable them to provide the support needed by students and staff.

Other studies have reported this lack of clinical teaching on the part of nurse teachers (Crotty, 1993; Crotty and Butterworth, 1992). For example, Crotty (1993), found that those nurse teachers who do maintain clinical contact, find that their role in this regard has become one of support for, and liaison with clinical nurses with little "hands on" work with students. Likewise, Jowett et al., (1994) give a similar picture of this attenuated clinical role, but also report that some nurse teachers also engage in ward based tutorials, discussions on learning objectives and the giving of feedback on written work. However, regarding such tutorials, one student commented:

> ...We did have someone [a teacher] come to a ward where there were a lot of heart operations and we were expecting something from them on that and we actually got a session on Parkinson's disease, so it seemed to be purely random.... (Jowett et al., 1994, p. 62).

The lack of clinical role clarity was also recognised by students in Davies, et al's (1996) study of Project 2000 nurse teachers' role in the clinical setting. The authors report how one student that they interviewed said:

> Its hard for them (tutors). I don't always have them (visits). I say 'I will contact you when I need you', because I feel it's a waste of time, because there's not really much they can help me with- apart from if I have a problem. But they are having difficulty finding their role (Davies et al, 1996, p. 23).

This was further accentuated whereby it became evident in this study that nurse teachers were having great difficulty defining their potential role in the clinical setting. The authors point out how these nurse teachers seemed to find this lack of clarity in relation to their role disconcerting. The majority of respondents indicated that they no longer perceived themselves as part of the ward team and felt that this restricted any influence they could exercise on clinical practice.

A number of models of clinical involvement have been proposed as being appropriate for enabling Project 2000 nurse teachers to maintain their clinical credibility. One such model, that of lecturer/practitioner, has received much attention in the literature (Kirk et al., 1997; Carlisle, et al., 1997; Rhead and Strange, 1996; Cave, 1994; Burnard and Chapman, 1990). Rhead and Strange (1996), both lecturer practitioners, advocate such a role as they maintain that it offers much to assist in decreasing the theory-practice gap. However, Cave (1994), in an analysis of the potential contribution of the lecturer-practitioner role and the link teacher role in assisting nurse teachers to maintain clinical credibility, concludes that the former is for a minority of teachers only and is not without its problems. Moreover, a number of other studies also demonstrate how the lecturer-practitioner role can overcome the theory-practice gap (Lathlean, 1992; Cowper, 1989; Wenban, 1985; Kings Fund, 1984 and Simons, 1984), this primarily due to the fact that in this role, the person who teaches must have clinical competence as they are also involved in clinical practice on a regular and sustained basis (typically 50% of their work time). Cave (1994) argues however, that while lecturer-practitioners can inform other teachers of the changes in clinical practice, there is a risk of recreating a divide between lecturer-practitioners and other teachers, similar to that which existed between nurse tutors and clinical teachers. The role that Cave advocates for the majority of nurse teachers therefore, is that of the link-teacher, suggesting that while this role does not confer the teacher with clinical competence, it does afford clinical credibility. In this role the teacher is not necessarily engaged in hands-on nursing care (indeed is unlikely to be so). Rather, she/he is in regular contact with clinical staff in a supportive and liaison capacity, and hence is aware of changes in clinical practice which subsequently can inform her/his teaching (Cave, 1994). Indeed, it would appear that this role is more akin to the role that many of the nurse teachers described in the studies discussed earlier. Unfortunately however, Cave goes on to report that the link-teacher role is not being adopted effectively. The chief reason for this failing is according to Kershaw (1990), the lack of funding to enable teachers adequate time to pursue this role. In conclusion, Cave warns that the role of the nurse tutor is being eroded by highly qualified specialists in Higher education, and by more knowledgeable, articulate practitioners. The author urges nurse teachers to develop sufficient clinical ability to be able to apply theory to current practice (Cave, 1994). Moreover, Carlisle, et al., (1997) warn of the difficulties that might arise should clinical teaching be left to clinical nurses alone, as was suggested to be the likely future situation by nurse teachers (n= 600) interviewed in the study. The authors draw attention to the current situation in the UK whereby clinical staff within the new market-led health service, with the potential for higher levels of autonomy they have within trusts, may well not see the clinical education of student nurses as a justifiable priority or responsibility. Furthermore, Davies et al., (1996) discovered that certain nurse teachers felt that some practitioners did not have the requisite knowledge or skills to enable students to make links between theory and practice. Conversely, some practitioners were not convinced of the clinical credibility of their teacher colleagues. The authors report that only some clinical nurses in the study had completed the ENB 998 course (Teaching and Assessing in Clinical Practice). Many practitioners it would seem were dependent upon short in-house courses, the main focus of which was on the interpretation and completion of assessment documentation.

Carlisle et al., (1997) also report that nurse teachers in their study suggested that while the desirable future situation is one whereby nurse teachers will engage in teaching clinical skills, and will work alongside students in delivering patient care, it was unlikely to materialise. While the respondents in this study suggested that some retention of clinical responsibility was necessary, and that part of that should primarily be as a practitioner and not as a teacher, many nurse teachers expressed a lack of confidence in their clinical skills. Further, it would appear that not everyone was in agreement in terms of nurse teachers having a clinical role. In this regard, one nurse teacher in Carlisle et al's (1997) study commented: "I actually had is said to me that I was no longer a nurse, I was a teacher now and that my role in the clinical area was as an education officer and facilitator." (Carlisle et al., 1997, p. 389).

The authors conclude that the time is right for nurse teachers to take a more proactive role in increasing their responsibility for the acquisition of clinical expertise among Project 2000 students (Carlisle et al., 1997).

1.8   Practical Placements

Project 2000 differs from the traditional programme in that it places more emphasis on health education, the prevention of ill health, and on community care. Therefore, earlier placements usually require students to spend some time observing the behaviour of healthy people before moving on to learn about caring for people who are ill. While initial practical experience placements are both in hospital and the community, there is a heavy weighting towards the latter in the Common Foundation Programme (CFP). The result of this new focus is that Project 2000 has become much more complex in terms of accessing and organising appropriate placements in a diversity of settings, many of which are not used to having student nurses on their premises (NAO, 1992). Moreover, it has also required the creation of a full time post of placements officer at most colleges.

According to the National Audit Office (1993), managers implementing Project 2000 have faced several difficulties. One such difficulty concerns the access to suitable placements for student nurses practical component of the course. It would appear that in some hospitals this proved difficult due to an inadequate skill mix, for example, where there were a high proportion of enrolled nurses and/or nursing assistants. In such a case, the NAO (1992) point out that the low proportion of registered nurses meant that there would not be enough qualified staff to act as mentors/preceptors as the few that were present would be too busy carrying out ward duties that only a registered nurse could do. Another problem concerns the difficulties that Project 2000 posed for the community services. Traditionally the community services were not accustomed to dealing with such a large number of student nurses. With the advent of Project 2000 and its strong community focus in the CFP, community services are finding themselves overstretched. A further complication is that the majority of the students placed in community settings are junior and hence require a significant amount of supervision. In the 10 sites visited by the NAO (1992), no provision had been made in the Project 2000 submissions to cost the implications of the new programme or to consider the extra resources required in community settings. The author cites the example of Hillingdon Community Unit who estimated that the additional annual cost during the Common Foundation Programme amounted to £130,000 out of a total budget of £4million. Another problem that occurred was that some community units had to release some registered nurses from the community sector to compensate for the service contribution made by the Project 2000 nurses. Indeed Jowett et al (1994) suggest that because of the scarcity of qualified staff, the problem of saturation of community areas with students is unlikely to abate in the near future. To an extent these difficulties limited the amount and diversity of practical experience available to students.

The NAO (1992) also reports how staff in all schemes made great efforts to organise appropriate placements. Innovative colleges established good relationships with local authorities and the private and voluntary sectors. For example, in the CFP, some had arranged placements in a diversity of settings such as shops, supermarkets, factories, railway stations, offices and department stores. Some minor difficulties have been reported with these ventures. For instance, some students on placements in supermarkets had been mistaken for shop assistants and asked to stack shelves, however, the NAO (1992) point out that such instances were easily ironed out by means of better communication. It would therefore appear that while reorientation to the community setting has been acknowledged and accepted as a required shift in thinking towards a changing health care focus, it is evident that the availability of resources and the level of planning will very much determine how successfully this can be achieved.

Other problems arose with the clinical supervision that was available. Jowett et al (1994) report that the amount of time required for the clinical teaching and supervision of the Project 2000 students is difficult to cope with when this is in addition to delivering patient care, particularly where placements are short and appropriate human resources are stretched. This was also recognised as a problem in one of the earlier studies of a demonstration district (Elkan et al 1993). In this study it was observed that even before the end of the first term it was accepted in principle by both ward and teaching staff that students could be included in performing basic tasks provided they received adequate supervision in the practice setting. Unfortunately however, this could not often be allowed as there were not always enough suitable qualified staff available to supervise the students. The authors report that almost all hospital and some community staff felt that they did not have the numbers of trained staff to supervise students properly (Elkan et al, 1993). Jowett et al (1994) report that there were marked differences between programmes regarding the extent to which sisters/charge nurses and second level registered nurses took on the role of mentor/supervisor. The authors report that in two of the demonstration districts, charge nurses or ward sisters did not normally adopt such a role, this primarily due to their ever increasing managerial responsibilities. All first-level registered nurses were eligible to act as supervisors after an initial settling in period for newly qualified staff. This was usually about six months, but was noted to be less in some instances. While it was against policy to do so, second level nurses were more likely to be engaged in student supervision. Further, the ideal of having one student per supervisor was unrealistic for many places and indeed there is evidence that the supervision commitment of some staff become somewhat of a burden (Jowett et al , 1994). Payne et al (1991) report how some nurse teachers had reservations about the level of preparedness and available support for clinical staff for their mentoring roles, and that they were not actively encouraged to develop such roles because of pressure of work and lack of resources. The authors continue:

> Time and again it seemed to some nurse teachers that clinical staff did not know what to do with the students'... nurse educators also worried that there were too few trained staff to take on the mentor roles (Payne et al., 1991, p. 16)

Spence (1994) points out that some clinical nurses are sceptical about Project 2000 and are lacking in confidence and understanding of their role with these students as they are too busy to familiarise themselves with the programme. Indeed, Casey (1996) argues that it is not realistic to expect clinical nurses who are products of the traditional programme to be able to embrace the philosophies of Project 2000 and the curriculum revolution just because they have been told about them. This is also evident from Elkan et al's (1993) study. The authors describe how in one placement area, there was a discrepancy in the goals of educators and those of clinical staff with regard to students self directed learning placement outcomes. They state: "thus, while the educationalists were trying to foster in students the qualities they deemed important for the nurse of the future, service staff were concerned more with the here and now task of producing safe, competent practitioners" (p. 37). This causes confusion for the students as it does not allow them to focus on or attain their specific placement outcomes, rather they are directed towards the "aims" of the ward staff. Casey (1996) suggests that the pressures to conform to socialisation in the practice setting are enormous. The student is often confused and has to choose between the values of the clinical staff and those that are emphasised in the classroom. Roles in practice areas are set out by senior nurses and by the practice setting itself. It is not easy for the student to resist the values and mores of the ward/placement.

There was also confusion among ward staff regarding the concept of supernumerary status (Elkan et al 1993; Payne et al., 1991).Payne and colleagues (1991) observe that the concept seemed to be widely misunderstood and that this was a considerable source of worry for nurse teachers, one of whom reported that some staff in practice areas seem to think that the new students would just stand and watch what was happening with their arms folded. Similarly Elkan et al (1993) report that both trained staff and even the students themselves were of the opinion that students were only to observe in their first two terms' placements. Hence, some students did just that, and qualified staff assumed they were correct in doing so. In other places however, this was interpreted by some staff as lack of interest on the part of the student.

Elkan et al (1993) noted that before long, and perhaps inevitably, comparisons in skill levels were being made between the new students and their traditional counterparts. The authors found that for nurse teachers, the development of clinical skills early in the CFP was not as important as the development of communication and interpersonal skills. On the contrary however, this was not the case for ward staff. Ward staff very much valued early skills acquisition and use this as a means to measure the relative worth of the student. The authors further expressed concern that teachers have placed so much emphasis on interpersonal skills and psychosocial care skills that the physical and manual skills are now relegated to a position of relative unimportance.

In 1994, Jowett et al noted considerable improvement in regard to students' practice placements. This the authors argue came about as a result of staff having had the opportunity to familiarise themselves more with the programme and with their role in this regard. Some respondents indicated that they felt that it was very much up to the students how much they benefited from their placements. Some students made it their business to get involved while others preferred to stand back. It would appear that the former group faired best from their placements. Jowett et al (1994) indicate that the students gave a varied and complex picture of the depth and extent of clinical supervision that they experienced. Even where the supervision arrangements were clearly inadequate however, the students did not necessarily feel that their learning had been compromised as a result. It was suggested that having other means of support often offset such inadequacies.

1.9 Calls for a Degree as the Sole Route of Entry

There have been many calls for an all graduate profession in the UK over the past 30 years or so. For example, in 1987 Baroness McFarlane of Llandaff made such a statement, suggesting that the future needs of the profession required graduate skills. The writer identifies developments such as primary nursing, clinical specialisation roles, nurse practitioner roles, as well as the need to develop nurses for management and research roles and the requirements for further development of nurse education as evidence of such a need. While McFarlane suggests that such a development is required by the year 2000, it would appear that in 1996, only 10% of student nurses in the UK were studying on degree courses (Willis, 1996).

Clarke and Warr (1995) question the morality of expecting student nurses to undertake a three year diploma programme whereby in order to upgrade to degree status (something that many employers are now asking for), they must undertake what for some is lengthy further studies. The authors argue that a degree is what should have been on offer in the first place, particularly as other health professionals are educated to graduate level. Project 2000 at diploma level is about preparation for practice the authors point out. Degree level education on the other hand prepares one for critical thinking, decision making, clinical judgement, and hence concerns education for practice. The authors comment:

> The new expectation for the year 2000 and beyond demands education to equip practitioners not just to be prepared, but to be able to be proactive in the practice of health care. This requires equal status with other decision makers. Diplomates are not graduates and therefore not equal (Clarke and Warr, 1995, p. 52).

Glasper and O'Connor (1996) suggest that a mistake was made during the Project 2000 negotiations that graduate status was not demanded by the profession. This the authors argue has left a legacy "that will bedevil and frustrate the efforts of those nurse educators seeking to embrace the twin philosophies of higher education, i.e. excellence in teaching and research." (p.5). The authors suggest that it is somewhat paradoxical, that at the very juncture when society was coming to the conclusion that to be a non-graduate was to be disenfranchised in the labour market, nurses decided to limit its higher education aspirations. The authors claim that many nurse academics from the United States and Australia consider the UK to be somewhat of an educational backwater because so few of its nurses are graduates. The authors, both of whom are nurse academics in higher education, conclude that nursing and midwifery will not be granted the respect given to other medical and paramedical professions until they achieve graduate status. Moreover, the authors argue, multidisciplinary working is dependent on a team of equals and hence equity within health care teams will require nurses and midwives who are graduates. In this regard, Castledine (1992) contends however, that nurses who are graduates will pose a threat to the status quo and to an entrenched health care system, one that has often been accused of being inadequate. The author argues that a key feature of the debate is to do with power and control. Educated nurses have power and usually cannot be easily controlled, the author concludes.

That pre-registration nurse education should be at degree level was also an issue that was recently debated by the Royal College of Nursing (RCN) (1997). Members of the College's Education and Training Policy Committee (ETPC) are of the opinion that nursing students should graduate at the point of entry to the profession. Furthermore, it has come to the attention of the committee that the present common foundation course is not compatible with European Union initiatives on the education and training of nurses. These initiatives concern a generalist model, this being proposed as it is believed to be the approach which will best serve the future health needs of the European people. Hence the RCN assert that the branch programmes are no longer an option if all nurses on the UK register are to be able to work freely in Europe. The ETPC conclude that a degree programme is now required for pre-registration nurse education in the UK and the committee has proposed such a structure moving through a pathway from preparation for entry to a degree programme, graduation and professional qualification. The RCN conclude that the Project 2000 diploma programme was developed to meet the healthcare needs in the year 2000. The proposed degree programme goes further, equipping the competent, professional practitioner with the necessary skills to integrate nursing practice with the work of other healthcare workers in order to meet the healthcare needs of a rapidly changing world (RCN, 1997).

Milligan (1997) at the end of a comprehensive literature review of pre-registration degree level education for nurses concludes that while such a move is probably inevitable, it is unclear however, when such a move will occur. Milligan notes from the literature, a number of proposed advantages of such a level of education, for example, improved quality of care given to clients, and the broadening of nurses roles in the future. The author suggests however that " apart from a clear statement in favour of pre-registration degree programmes by the RCN in 1996, there appears to be little desire to overtly support such moves at this time by either the UKCC or the ENB" (Milligan, 1997, p. 2).

Summary

Nursing in the United Kingdom has a long history of links with the higher education sector spanning most of this century. It also has had pre-registration degree programmes on offer in various universities for over thirty years now. However, until recently, these programmes have been for a select few. A plethora of myths about graduate nurses are evident in the literature. At the time of their inception, it was generally reported that graduates of these programmes would not enter nursing practice, or if they did, that they would not stay in clinical nursing. Furthermore, there was also the belief that those who did enter clinical practice, would be fast-tracked to management and senior education positions. This has not been the case. A number of outcome studies of nurse graduates have consistently shown that the exact opposite is the case. It appears that graduates not alone take up clinical nursing positions, but that they generally remain in these positions for many years. What has been shown however, is that graduate nurses tend to work in nursing posts that afford them greater autonomy, such as midwifery and community nursing.

A number of government reports have focused on nursing education in the United Kingdom over the past 50 years or so. Many of them drew attention to the problems of having student nurses as part of the workforce, arguing that student nurse training should be dictated by the learning needs of students rather than by the staffing needs of the hospital. Despite these reports, substantial change in the preparation of student nurses for professional practice did not come about until the late 1980s when the Department of Health declared it's broad acceptance of the UKCCs (1987) Project 2000 proposals. Indeed for some, this was a mistake, as many felt that graduate status was now required for nurses on entry to practice, if nursing was going to be able to meet the needs of the British population into the next millennium. Notwithstanding this, Project 2000 represented a major shift in thinking in the education of students for the nursing profession of the 1990s and beyond. The main aims of the programme were to produce a knowledgeable doer, a nurse who is capable of critical-analytical thinking, who can explain and justify practice that is based on a sound theoretical grounding, who can practice autonomously, and who can demonstrate professional accountability and commitment to continuing professional education. Indeed, the earliest outcome studies suggested that the new curriculum was making a positive impact on nursing practice. While it would appear that students were initially lacking in confidence and in clinical skills, evidence is it did not take long for them to catch up with their traditional counterparts. It is also evident from the outcome studies that many Project 2000 prepared nurses had a good depth of knowledge, adopted a more holistic approach to care, were less inclined to adhere to routines, displayed evidence of analytical decision-making skills, were confident interpersonally, and had highly developed academic skills.

The funding of Project 2000 was not without it's problems. The original Department of Health formula for estimating staff replacement costs was evidently flawed primarily because the entire structure on which the calculations were based subsequently became obsolete as a result of the gamut of changes that occurred during the NHS reforms. It has also been suggested that many of the components of the formula were based on unproved assumptions. There were also problems in the manner in which these monies were distributed at a local level.

There is both anecdotal and empirical evidence to suggest that student funding on Project 2000 courses is also lacking. Project 2000 students receive a non-means tested bursary, and they are exempt from income tax, national insurance and superannuation contributions, and they only have to pay 20% of their community charge (poll tax). Despite this, there are numerous reports in the nursing popular press of the United Kingdom, (some by national nurse leaders), suggesting that many students are living below the poverty line, and that they must rely on parental assistance or part-time low paid jobs in order to make ends meet.

Project 2000 heralded enormous changes also for nurse teachers. Of immediate concern was the need to attain graduate status. This goal was not alone a requirement of the ENB, but was also seen as being necessary if nurse teachers were to have academic credibility in the eyes of their higher education counterparts. What is evident is that many nurse teachers came under great pressure in pursuing this goal. Furthermore, there appears to have been a lack of direction as to what degree to pursue, and many had to study part-time, plan the new curriculum, as well as hold down a full-time job, all at the same time. In some places it is reported that too many nurse teachers were attending college at once with the result that there were insufficient numbers left behind to do the work.

Project 2000 also meant a change in teaching focus for many. While there is no doubt that many nurse teachers were already adopting a student centred learning approach, not all teachers were willing to embrace such principles of the new curriculum. The size of Project 2000 intakes and the lack of enough rooms in which to teach them sometimes thwarted attempts to adopt more student-centred approaches. Many Project 2000 teachers report a vast increase in their workload, not alone as a result of their need to read for degrees, but also due to the pressures they were now experiencing in having to engage in scholarly activity such as research and publications. It would also appear that due to the short lead in time, many schools were planning the Branch Programme long after the Common Foundation Programme had commenced. Another pressure impinging on nurse teachers was that of the need to develop clinical credibility. Indeed, nurse teachers were very much divided on this issue. Some felt that clinical work was central to and vital for their role as nurse teachers. Others expressed the view that they were now teachers and as such had no role in clinical activity. A number of models of clinical practice for nurse teachers are described in the literature, principally those of the lecturer-practitioner, and the link teacher.

While the diploma in higher education course, Project 2000, is still the most common route to registration as a nurse, an increasing number of nursing students are opting for pre-registration degree programmes. Moreover, there have been recent calls from a number of sources including the Royal College of Nursing, that this route should become the exclusive route to registration as a nurse. The main rationale for such calls are that Project 2000 is no longer seen to be an appropriate method of preparing nurses for the future health needs of the nation. There have also been suggestions that students on Project 2000 courses have already a sufficient amount and depth of study to warrant a degree (Wainwright, 1996). While the nature and extent of the links with higher education have varied considerably over the years since the inception of Project 2000, pre-registration nurse education is now fully integrated into the higher education sector (Hughes, 1998, personal communication).

CHAPTER 2

CHANGES IN NURSE EDUCATION – AUSTRALIA

2.1 A Brief History of Nurse Education

Australian nursing, like nursing in many of the other commonwealth countries, was originally based on the Nightingale model. This model was first introduced to the continent at the Sydney Infirmary by Lucy Osburn in 1872 (Harloe, et al., 1995) after the then Colonial Secretary of New South Wales, Sir Henry Parkes, had written to Florence Nightingale, requesting that she send some trained nurses to work at the Sydney Infirmary (National Review of Nurse Education, 1994). Shortly after taking up the post of Lady Superintendent at the hospital, Ms. Osburn established and personally supervised a nurse training school. Over the next few decades, Nightingale's philosophies and standards were adopted by the other states, and quickly spread throughout Australia. Many of the matrons of these hospitals came from among the original probationers trained by Osburn, while others were appointed directly from Britain (Russell, 1990; Wood, 1990). Despite Nightingale's outstanding research record and her expertise in the area of statistics, she did not emphasise these activities in nursing education of the time (Smith, 1982). Rather, nursing education in Australia at the end of the nineteenth century followed an identical model to that used in Britain. This was described by Russell (1990), as one that was specifically structured in order to ensure conformity, obedience and high standards of care, but not independent analytical thinking or assertiveness on the part of the nurse. Russell (1990) points out how students were carefully selected by the matron on the basis of both their educational and their moral standards. Vocational training, board, lodging and uniforms were then provided at no cost, and the students received a meagre wage. In return for their training, students were expected to cater for the service needs of the hospital. Student nurses alternated through specific clinical areas to obtain experience under the direction of the ward sister' in each area. It was considered necessary that the ward sisters should themselves be qualified nurses who were both able and willing to teach and supervise the student nurses. Russell (1990) argues that this arrangement is similar to that of an apprenticeship, in which the artisan or master craftsman teaches the apprentice a trade or craft.

This model of nursing remained for the greater part unchanged for the next century (1872-1980s), and indeed, according to the National Review on Nurse Education (1994), is still evident in Australian nurse education. So much so is this the case, that Russell (1990) argues that there are still many nurses who continue to resist any attempts to change this situation. Indeed it will be seen in this chapter how early attempts during the

1930s to move nurse education into the tertiary education sector failed due to staunch resistance from within the profession itself (Harloe, et al., 1995). According to the National Review (1994), the Nightingale model remained popular in Australia for so long, primarily as it continued to meet workforce needs at a time when hospitals were expanding rapidly throughout Australia. Furthermore, like elsewhere, this model was seen as one that had great potential to advance the professionalisation of nursing at the time.

2.2 The Gradual Move towards University Based Pre-registration Nurse Education

History of Nurse Education

At the turn of this century, all State health authorities employed student nurses as part of their workforce, however, it was up to individual hospitals to decide on the nature and extent of the programme of training that they offered to students. Further, funding for nurse education was provided from each individual hospital's budget (National Review, 1994). Invariably, this lead to a wide diversity of different programmes, and the quality of nurse education was totally dependent upon the importance placed on it by each hospital's board of management (Wood, 1990). That each hospitals curriculum for nurse education varied is well illustrated by Forsyth, (1995), an in particular, the central role played by the medical profession, and the control they exercised over nurse education at that time is summed up by that author's comment:

> The training of student nurses at the outset, although formally under the auspices of the matron, was in practice controlled by the senior doctors who had influence over both the content and the delivery of the nursing curriculum. Decisions concerning the curriculum, and any structural changes to it always had to be ratified by the board. In this way, the board and its members regulated nursing knowledge and practice (Forsyth, 1995, p. 167).

Indeed, the author further points out how as the curriculum became more organised, the involvement of the medical profession increased and in 1888, the board put forward changes to the curriculum: "embodying concise teaching upon every subject with which a nurse should be acquainted...without embarrassing them with unnecessary knowledge." (Annual Report, 1888, p. 8. cited in Forsyth, 1995).

In 1899, a number of leading nursing and medical personnel established the New South Wales, Trained Nurses Association, which later that year changed its name to the Australian Trained Nurses Association (ATNA). Before long, branches of the association were established throughout the other states, and agreement was reached that members of one could transfer at ease to another. Russell (1990) points out how membership of these associations quickly became an important status symbol for nurses. Among their aims were the establishment of a minimal standard of education for nurses, the maintenance of a nurses register, the accreditation of schools of nursing for training student nurses, and the approval of the nominations of matrons for hospitals receiving a government subsidy. This was an important achievement as it meant that for the first time nurse education was organised in Australia at a national level, with admission to the nursing register controlled by a State-wide examination. In 1924 however, the Nurses Registration Act was passed and therefore the responsibility of registering nurses fell to the State Government. However, several key members of the ATNA were appointed to the first Nurses Registration Board, so effectively, nurses maintained considerable control over nurse training (Russell, 1990; 1992).

The Need for Change

The period between the 1930s and the 1980s was one of continual agitation by nurses for educational reform during which time the old system of nurse preparation came under much pressure. Much of the discontent with the traditional system came about as a result of a number of factors that primarily concerned both the status of nursing *vis a vis* that of other health professionals, and also, the poor pay and conditions that nurses had to endure. Another issue of concern was the high attrition rates among nurses, which in part at least, was linked to the two factors mentioned above.

A plethora of official reports were produced over the years, the express aims of which were to address these and other issues concerning the education of nurses. For instance, Wood (1990) reports that the Kelly Committee (1943) found nurse training to be unsatisfactory and therefore recommended that it be replaced with a system of education that was grounded in sound educational principles and which would provide nurses who were capable of serving the needs of the Australian people into the next decades. Similarly, in 1967, a committee on nursing in New South Wales suggested that student nurses were being prepared too quickly for ward duties and as a result were not receiving the required theoretical instruction, the result of which was that these nurses were restricted in their outlook, resistant to change, and unable to cope confidently with the scientific and technical advances in medicine. What was needed the authors argued, was a programme of study which would "enable the interest of the intelligent student to be maintained....[and which would] encourage critical thinking and develop potential." (Institute of Hospital Matrons, cited in Sax, 1978, p. 10). Wood (1990) indicated that by the early 1970s there was wide agreement in New South Wales that there was a need for higher standards in nurse education and also, that the time was ripe to move nurse education from its traditional hospital base. The National Review (1994) suggest that the options that emerged in place of hospital training schools were university based education, colleges of advanced education, and regional schools of nursing. A significant step towards university based education came in 1970 when the Minister of Health advocated that these latter two venues be given responsibility for certificate or diploma courses leading to registration while the universities would extend the few combined degree programmes that had been established since the late 1960s (National Review, 1994). In 1967 the University of New England (UNE) commenced a combined nurse training course with an Arts degree in association with two teaching hospitals. There followed a similar course in 1968 at the University of New South Wales. Russell (1990) suggests that these departures were very much influenced by similar ventures overseas, particularly in the UK, and that like their counterparts in the UK, the courses were designed to serve a minority of nurses, principally those with greater than average academic ability.

In addition to those dealing specifically with nursing and nurse education, there were a number of other reports on hospitals and on health services in general that were published during this period (Russell, 1988). These reports examined a variety of issues concerning health care such as labour force planning, funding, and rationalisation of existing services. Russell points out that because nurses represented a large proportion of the health workforce, most if not all of these reports gave some consideration to nursing and/or nurse education. At an international level, a number of other bodies were examining nurse education, this principally as a result of the recommendations of the World Health Organisation Expert Committee on Nursing (1966). In this regard, Shorten and McMurray (1992) suggest that developments in North America also served as an impetus for educational reform in Australia. In particular, a number of measures that were introduced to improve the standard of the pre-registration nursing courses in these two countries lead to a situation whereby the Australian nurse qualification was no longer acceptable for work in these countries. Instead, Australian nurses who wished to work in the UK and USA were now required to gain additional clinical experience (Russell, 1988). The author continues, that the inability to obtain registration abroad was seen as a further example of the perceived inferiority of the Australian nursing education system.

According to Russell (1988), the findings of these official reports represented a severe incrimination of nurse training and graphically emphasised many of the woes that beset nursing at the time. In particular, the reports revealed that there was a lack of suitable recruits for nursing principally due to a poor educational standard, and also that there was an unacceptably high attrition rate among nursing students, the result of which was a shortage of nurses with which to staff the hospital system (Truskett Report, 1971 cited in Russell, 1988). Of further concern was the finding that many did not practice as nurses on completion of training (Kelly Report, 1967 cited in Russell, 1988). The major reasons given by nurses for not working in the hospital sector were poor remuneration, disruption to social life caused by shift work, and the unco-operative attitude of hospital administrators (Russell, 1988). Regarding problems relating to the mode of educational preparation, Russell (1988) identifies a number of other factors that were critical in propelling moves towards change. These included that the apprenticeship model lead to a situation whereby service needs took precedence over students learning needs, a lack of correlation between theory and practice and, a lack of suitably qualified nurse teachers. Similarly, Happell (1996) suggests that for many years preceding the eventual move of nurse education to the tertiary sector, nursing education was seen as deficient in five main areas as outlined in Table 2.1

TABLE 2.1.   Perceived deficiencies in nurse education

- It maintained the subservient position of nurses in relation to other health professionals, most notably doctors.
- The focus of hospital-based education was narrow and restrictive and provided little scope for critical awareness and reflective thinking.
- Nurses were denied true student status.
- There was an inadequate relationship between theory and practice.
- Hospital-based education was viewed as an inappropriate venue for facilitating the changing role of the nurse in view of changes in technology and the focus of care.

Source adapted from: **Happell, 1996, p. 112.**

The main means of addressing these issues were according to Happell (1996), the adoption of a curriculum with a comprehensive knowledge base and a reduction in the predominance of the medical model, the awarding of full student status and, an increase in the correlation between theory and practice and better responsiveness to the ongoing changes in the role of the nurse.

Other critics of the traditional system expressed concern with the situation of nurse education in the clinical settings. For example, Russell (1990) commented that the learning experiences of student nurses in the clinical areas were for the greater part unstructured and somewhat hit and miss. This was primarily due to the fact that all too often the service role was seen to take precedence over the learning role, and also due to the long-standing situation whereby funding for nurse education very much depended on the disposition of the budget-holding lay administrators. Moreover, the National Review (1994) pointed out how the apprenticeship system became one of the prominent political questions of the day in regard to its ability to prepare nurses for a changing Australia, one with an ever increasingly complex and technological system of health provision, and also for a situation whereby the future shape of the Australian population was set to change rapidly, with consequential changes in health needs. The conclusions of these expert committees demonstrated considerable agreement about the actual problems that beleaguered nursing education. However, nursing in Australia at this time (early 1970s) did not speak with a single unifying voice. There were many nursing organisations, none of which spoke for the majority of the profession. However, in 1973, primarily in response to government inaction, a working party with representatives from all of the major nursing organisations was established with the express aim of developing clear goals in nursing education (Russell, 1988). This was a significant departure, as now, for the first time, the might of nursing spoke with one voice, and this unprecedented happening, was clearly intimidating to politicians and health service managers (National Review, 1994). The steering committee which was set up as a result of this liaison became a significant pressure group in improving nursing education, and in expediting its transfer to the tertiary sector (Russell, 1988).

Proposals for change were not without their detractors. Russell (1988 & 1990) points out how the traditional system of nurse preparation had stood the test of time and in general was seen to have met the needs of the healthcare system. This is of course a valid argument, however, such a model is unlikely to continue to meet those needs due to the aforementioned unprecedented changes in the healthcare requirements of the Australian population. Concerns were also expressed that any such changes in nurse education would reduce the number of applicants thereby exacerbating nursing shortages.[1] This concern was voiced on the pretext that if nurse education moved to the tertiary sector, then the Higher School Certificate would become the standard of entry and hence, the number of applicants would be reduced. This it was felt would result in a crisis situation for many hospitals as student nurses provided between 60 to 80 percent of direct patient care (National Review of Nurse Education, 1994).

Objections were also voiced by the medical profession, and paramount in the thinking of hospital administrators and politicians were concerns regarding the cost implications of such changes (Harloe et al., 1995; Russell, 1988). Indeed, Marquis, et al., (1993) point out that perhaps the greatest stumbling block was to do with funding.

Nursing education in hospitals was traditionally funded through the health budget. If moved to higher education however, funding would become a part of the education budget. The authors go on to explain how the catalyst to begin the move that would ultimately lead to the transfer came about as a result of political manoeuvring in the heavily populated state of New South Wales. This state was at the time facing a funding crisis in health care. The authors point out that moving nursing from the health budget to the education budget would resolve the dilemma. The authors continue: "The political

---

[1] In some States, up to 50% of students dropped out of training before completing the course (National Review of Nurse Education, 1994).

actions in New South Wales, combined with increased pressure from all nursing groups, forced the federal government to address the question." (Marquis et al., 1993, p. 136).

One final report was instrumental in paving the way for substantial educational change. In 1978, the report of the Commonwealth Tertiary Education Commission's Committee of Inquiry into Nurse Training and Education (Sax Report), stated that the development of the necessary skills for professional nursing practice requires a more academic approach to be adopted in nurse education. Despite the fact that the committee sat at a period of great pressure from nursing organisations, their conclusion was that this recommendation could be effectively addressed within an upgraded hospital training system (National Review, 1994). However, the committee did recommend that hospitals should form alliances with tertiary establishments and that they could seek accreditation for courses at advanced educational level. Furthermore, it recommended that such advanced courses be permitted to extend to 2200 places (about 10% of all student nurse places). The overall objective of this report was according to the National Review (1994) to situate pre-registration nurse education at diploma level, with provision for diplomates to advance to bachelor degree level at a later date.

Needless to say, the nursing profession was on the whole disappointed with the report and its failure to adequately situate nurse education in the tertiary sector (Russell, 1990). However, a further blow was dealt by the commonwealth governments abject refusal to support even a moderate expansion of nurse education into the higher education sector (National Review, 1994). There followed in 1983 a series of workshops, instigated by the various nursing organisations, to review the situation, and it was determined that the more appropriate academic award for completion of the pre-registration nurse education programme was a Bachelor of Applied Science Degree in Nursing and not the recommended diploma (Wood, 1990). This came at a critical period as these workshops immediately preceded the 1983 Federal Elections.

As part of its election manifesto, the Labour Party declared that it would establish 2200 nursing places in advanced education by 1985 as recommended by the Sax Report (1978). However, soon after the election, it became apparent that the newly elected government might be persuaded to go even further than this (National Review, 1994). An initial proposal was made by the new Government for a three year diploma to be taught in colleges of advanced education with clinical instruction to be conducted in specified hospitals attached to each college. The National Review (1994) recounts how on 11th May, 1984, the Sax Report was symbolically burned at a national conference of nurses in Adelaide as a result of the publication earlier that day of a government report that failed to once and for all, situate nurse education in the higher education sector. There followed a series of other committee investigations of the nursing case, and on 24th August, 1984, the Commonwealth Government announced its in-principle support for the full transfer of registered nurse preparation to the higher education sector, a feat that was to be completed by the end of 1993. The standard qualification was to be a three-year diploma, with part of the students course time spent in a diversity of health care settings.

2.3   The Transfer to Higher Education

The Significance of the Move

The decision to transfer pre-registration nurse education to the higher education sector in 1984 was a monumental and courageous undertaking according to Bennett (1996), and one that had major implications for nursing, and for the nature of nursing work (National Review, 1994). However, whilst welcoming the transfer, Madjar, (1995) laments the fact that Australian nursing education gained entry into universities "at least in part, as a result of political concerns with economies of scale'..." (p. 129). Nonetheless, as evidenced from the previous section, the decision was the culmination of many years of hard work, planning and exertion of political pressure on the part of the nursing profession. The move signified many things for many people, chief among which was that it represented a modernised education system which would be better resourced, would provide a broader knowledge base and an opportunity for autonomous learning. It would not alone ensure that all nurses of the future would be adequately prepared for beginning nursing practice, but also that it would set the seeds for the preparation of advanced practitioners for all areas of nursing (Bennett, 1996; Hart, 1985). All of this, it was hoped, would lead to more autonomous and professional nursing practice. Indeed the hopes of many nurses that these changes would bring about such results, is well summed up by Bennett's comment:

> Graduates of the programmes would be competent practitioners equipped with the appropriate knowledge, skills and attitudes to not only provide quality nursing care but also shape the healthcare system into the next century (Bennett, 1996, p. 3).

In addition the author argues, the direction of nursing programmes in the university setting would assist the development of the discipline of nursing through its fostering of both research and other academic activity, the result of which would be the generation of knowledge that would enhance both the practice and knowledge base of nursing (Bennett, 1996). However, Madjar, (1995) suggests that the sense of a nursing research culture is only beginning to emerge in Australia and warns that this situation is further compounded by a lack of research degrees in nursing, the result of which is that staff often end up conducting research within other disciplines. In this regard, the author comments:

> We will not make a significant contribution to the development of our own discipline, nor to the development of a local culture of nursing research while our energies are dissipated in too many different directions (Madjar, 1995, p. 130).

Despite all the changes that have occurred in Australian nursing over the past century, and in particular, despite the fact that nurses themselves have embraced the changes in education in order to develop and increase their body of knowledge and improve nursing practice, little has changed regarding the image of nursing according to Dahl (1992). The author, a second year nursing degree student, observes that the traditional image of nursing as an occupation that is subservient to medicine and lay administration, has yet to change. This is a view also propounded by Forsyth (1995) in her treatise on the historical continuities and constraints in the professionalisation of nursing. In her paper, the author catalogues a series of controls that were placed upon the nursing profession over the years, principally by the medical profession and by the state. The author concludes that these influences still survive today, suggesting that the main problem confronting contemporary nursing is that its capability to professionalise continues to be constrained by the state, thus demonstrating an historical continuity with the past.

The Transfer Process

The transfer of pre-registration nursing education into the tertiary sector coincided with a period of rationalisation and major change in the higher education sector. These changes included a major expansion in enrolments, the abolition of the old colleges of advanced education and hence an end to the binary system, and a greater emphasis on accountability and quality management. Further, it would also appear that nursing entered the tertiary sector at a time of rapid deterioration in funding levels per student. As a result, the arrival of nursing in higher education at this time was welcomed by many institutions as it facilitated their development in terms of offering them a new source of enrolments (National Review, 1994). Indeed, Marquis et al., (1993) argue that because departments of nursing brought with them large numbers of students, and as a consequence, increased funding, they were willingly accommodated by university and college administrators. Prior to this the authors argue, nursing was only extended a token acceptance from their new hosts.

The pace and scale of change brought with it both problems and opportunities for nursing. The number of institutions offering pre-registration nurse education was being halved and the number of students increased by 40% over five years, thus the initial passage of nursing to the higher education sector was eased. Conversely, with the rules of the game constantly shifting, the transfer became a more intricate operation (National Review, 1994). According to the Review, the professional education of nurses was not alone moving to higher education, but also, it was being transformed from an advanced education discipline to a university discipline, and as will become clear later in this discourse, from diploma status to degree status. Despite the fact that the culture of the Colleges of Advanced Education was closely related to that of the universities, nevertheless, the result of this colossal transfer was that some nurses, in particular nurse educators, suffered from varying degrees of culture shock, and regrettably in some cases, the theory-practice gap widened. Indeed, these were not easy times in which to try to establish a new university discipline (Madjar, 1995).

Despite the foregoing, the net result of the transfer was generally held to have been positive (Bennett, 1996; Forsyth, 1995; National Review, 1994; Marquis, et al., 1993; Hart, 1985). The opportunities offered by the universities, for both research and other scholarly activity were particularly welcomed, while Hart (1985) suggests that the university location also confirms that nursing had achieved unambiguous status as a profession alongside other long established professions. Moreover, the National Review (1994) argues that the opportunity for nurses to enter into university studies in their own discipline, up to doctoral level, opens up new possibilities for development, not alone for the individual nurse, but also for the profession and for the health services as a whole.

The joint ministerial statement of 24th August 1984 confirmed that implementation of the transfer of nursing education into the higher education domain was dependent on the outcome of negotiations regarding cost-sharing and transition arrangements with each of the states and territories. According to the agreed terms, the States and Territories undertook to provide 75% of recurrent expenditure and all capital expenditure associated with pre-registration nurse education for the duration of the transfer period (1985-1993) (National Review, 1994). Under the States Grants (Nurse Education Assistance) Act 1985, the Commonwealth Government was liable to meet the remaining 25% of recurrent funding. Furthermore, the total number of student places sanctioned at the outset was 18,000 equivalent full-time students. Also, the States agreed to transfer only on the provision that the cost would be no more than those accrued in the traditional system. It was later agreed that as and from 1994, basic nurse education would be funded in the

50

same way that other higher education places were, in other words, the Commonwealth would take over all funding (National Review, 1994).

There was marked variation among states in terms of the timing of the transfer process. For example, New South Wales had opted for the transfer in principle almost a year before the Commonwealth announcement and moved quickly, thus completing the process in one year. Moreover, Victoria proceeded more gradually in order to assist in the management of the process in both the health and education sectors. In each region of Victoria, one hospital-based programme was maintained after others had been phased out, so that the supply of registered nurses was safeguarded. Furthermore, there was also considerable variation in the actual number of places filled compared with those originally sanctioned. In Western Australia, the number of places was exactly as planned, however, in New South Wales and Queensland, a reduced number of places were offered, while Victoria offered an increased number of places.

At the time of the transfer period, the overall agreed student intake consisted of the agreed jointly funded intakes plus extra places which were funded by individual states in order to enable them to meet perceived demand for new registered nurses. There were also a few pilot scheme places (N= 1800) and these were funded by the Commonwealth. However, in the latter 1980s, it transpired that there was a shortage of nurses and therefore state funded places were increased where necessary. Indeed, in Victoria, some of the old traditional schools were temporarily re-opened for this reason. On the whole, actual student numbers during the transfer period were higher than had been anticipated in 1985. In fact, the Department of Employment, Education and Training (DEET) figures demonstrate that the number of pre-registration higher education nursing students grew by more than 30,000 during the period of the transfer, this representing an increase in nursing's share of total health science places in the tertiary education sector from 8% in 1984, to more than 30% in 1990. In terms of overall higher education places, nursing increased from 0.4% in 1984 to 5.3% in 1990 and 6.2% in 1993. (National Review, 1994). This development is particularly interesting in that initially, there was considerable concern that in fact colleges and universities would be unable to attract enough recruits into nursing to meet demand. Further, the advent of a nursing strike in Victoria, and the shortages in available registered nurses in 1996 compounded these fears (Marquis et al, 1993). The authors go on to point out that while these shortages were not the result of the loss of student labour as a result of the transfer, the situation was capitalised upon by those who were opposed to the transfer. While it is reported that most nurses publicly supported the need for college based nursing education and were committed to accomplishing the goals of the transfer, some regarded nurse academics as ex-nurses and felt that the transfer would result in a dilution of clinical nursing skills (Mason, 1991a). Moreover, Madjar (1995) voices her concern that nursing, by entering the tertiary sector, may be doing little more than "trading the very soul of nursing in exchange for the academic status for a select few." (p. 129). She postulates that being in the academic world may in fact represent a withdrawal from the problems and realities of practice into the ivory towers of esoteric theories. If managed properly however, the author suggests that higher education may have much to offer nursing stating that: "It is the combination of sound formal education and reflective practice in a collegial atmosphere which is most likely to produce expert practitioners, ..." (Madjar, 1995, p. 129).

In 1987, some doctors and politicians proposed a dual system of education for nurses. This was based upon the rationale that retaining hospital-based training programmes as well as the addition of college programmes would offer more choice to nurses, and also, would produce an adequate numbers of nurses to meet service needs. The public outcry and series of demonstrations that followed were un precedented according to Marquis et al (1993). The authors describe how nurses marched through the streets of Sydney in protest, calling for the immediate and complete transfer of nursing education to the tertiary sector. The final platform for the move to higher education was now set and a comment by Lumby in 1989 echoed the sentiments of many Australian nurses at this time:

> The professionalisation of Australian nurses is now in its final stages. Freed from the complex accountability dictated by the apprenticeship model of education, and without the constraints of bureaucracy, the standard of relationship between student and client may be more freely dictated by the profession and the professional (Lumby, 1989, p. 292).

Upgrading to Degree Status

By 1989, the advanced education sector was abolished and was replaced with what became known as the Unified National System of higher education. At about this time, Australian universities began to phase out sub-bachelor diploma courses and began to integrate them with existing degree programmes or converting them to new degree programmes. As a result, the integrity of diploma courses from the advanced education sector was called into question (National Review, 1994). The following year, both on the advice of the Commonwealth minister for Employment, Education and Training, and as a result of pressure from within the nursing profession itself, the Australian Educational Council agreed that the initial qualification for registered nurses should be a three year (six semester) bachelors degree, and that this should be achieved by 1992. It would appear that there were some calls for a four degree, however, these were largely unsuccessful. One problem with this arrangement however, was that funding for the degree remained at the same level as that for the diploma (National Review, 1994).

According to Marquis et al., (1993) this new departure to degree status had a marked effect on academe, and on society as a whole. In Australia, bachelor's degrees in nursing are usually applied science degrees. This differs from the situation in the United States of America where nursing degrees are usually bachelor of science degrees. The significance of this difference is that in Australia therefore, science courses are usually developed specifically for nursing students. The off-side of this however is that as a result, students often do not get to integrate into campus life as they are very much educated in isolation from students from other disciplines.

There were also other difficulties with nursing's new found degree status. One such difficulty is that cited by Marquis (1988) whereby the author argues that some aspects of Australian society was not yet ready to accept such a new image of nursing. In States that initially continued to offer limited traditional hospital training schools, there was frequently competition to gain admittance before these schools closed. The author describes how some parents expressed the view that their daughters could only hope to become a "real" nurse if they could secure a place on one of the few remaining traditional courses. Indeed Harvey (1988) in a paper describing her experiences on graduating as a nurse, describes how she encountered "mixed attitudes" from existing registered nurses, other health carers, and from the general public. Much of this the author contends came about as a result of ignorance on their part, regarding the nature of the new programme of study. Concerns were also expressed that the transfer of nursing into higher education would result in a situation whereby the profile of entrants into nursing would change, and that it would begin to reflect the socio-economic bias generally evident in higher education, thus discouraging participation by certain groups (South Australia Health

52

Commission, 1986). Neil and Barclay (1989) for this reason advocate that such sociodemographic studies need to be undertaken as a matter of urgency in Australian nursing. Moreover, the authors cite a study by Wright (1988) who found that college nursing programmes in New South Wales, contrary to the generally held belief, increased recruitment across all socio-economic levels and thus broadened nursing's entry base. A limitation to this however, is that no details are given about how this finding was arrived at.

Whilst acknowledging that there have been some problems with the new degree programme, not least the disagreements regarding the appropriate duration of such a course, Marquis et al., (1993) contend that Australia has taken a giant step towards the systematic organisation of nurse education and the professionalisation of nursing. The authors conclude that there is a certain level of confidence in the profession that the new approach to nurse education will ensure that Australian nursing will be at the forefront of developments in both nursing practice and academy into the 21st century, not alone in the Pacific Rim countries, but also at an international level.

In 1993, the vast majority of pre-registration student nurses were enrolled on bachelor's degree programmes, most diploma programmes having being phased out by now. In, 1994 there were 28 higher education institutions in Australia offering nursing courses (National Review, 1994). While nursing at this time, constituted 7.2% of Australia's undergraduate student force, it constituted only 0.3% of PhD students and 0.8% of those pursuing research masters programmes.

2.4   Structure of the Pre-registration Undergraduate Programme

Curriculum Model

Pre-registration undergraduate nurse education programmes in Australia follow a generalist model whereby at the end of the programme, students are qualified to work in variety of practice settings such as general nursing, mental health nursing, children's nursing, elderly care, and community nursing, among others (Farrell and Carr, 1996; National Review, 1994). The rationale for adopting such a model stemmed principally from the view that this type of programme would provide a broad based flexible approach which would best meet the needs of the future health of the Australian people, however, fiscal motives were also implicated (National Review, 1994). Midwifery is not included in this generalist model, rather programmes that lead to a midwifery registration are at a post-graduate/post-registration level. Regarding such an approach, the World Health Organisation (1994) suggest that with refinement of skills through supervision, a generalist nurse should be able to provide for the physical and mental health needs of the client, and that a generalist perspective suggests that discipline maturity occurs after registration. Previously, separate undergraduate level courses in specialist areas such as children's nursing and mental health nursing, were offered, however, this mode of preparation was phased out in the early to mid 1990s, and since then all of these specialities have been subsumed into the generalist degree programme. Indeed in Australia, a number of specialist education programmes, including those that form strands in the generalist pre-registration programmes such as mental health, are offered at a post-graduate level.

Notwithstanding the benefits that were suggested of adopting a generalist curriculum model, this approach was not without its problems. Farrell and Carr (1996) identified all universities in Australia that had schools of nursing (N=32) and contacted the Heads of

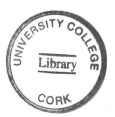

Department of these schools requesting information on the mental health component of the pre-registration undergraduate nursing programme. The researchers sent a postal questionnaire to all of these individuals requesting their help in documenting the number of theoretical hours devoted to a "mental illness focus" which was defined as: "curricula that include, for example, an introduction to mental disorder; the psychology of abnormal behaviour; and nursing interventions for patients with a mental disorder" (p.79-79). Respondents (n=26, response rate 84%) were also asked to document the amount of hours that students were placed in mental health clinical settings. The authors discovered that the number of theoretical hours varied considerably from 0 to 225 (M= 75, SD= 57), while those in practicum ranged from 0 to 200 hours (M=92, SD= 59). Schools registering shorter theory hours were not necessarily those with shorter practice hours. The researchers conclude that students could graduate and progress immediately to work in mental health settings with little or no practical and/or theoretical learning in the specialist area of mental health (Farrell and Carr, 1996). While this writer has no evidence of the same situation pertaining in any of the other strands to the generalist programme, the possibility of this occurring cannot be discounted.

The possibility of a common core approach to the nursing curriculum was also discussed at length in the National Review (1994). First of all, the issue of a common core within nursing curricula where a national framework governing such issues as the length of courses, the course structure, and course content would be established, was considered. The Review reports that there was strong opposition to the idea of standardisation of course structure and content, however, the majority were in favour of a standard length, the preferred length being four years. A common core within the health sciences was also considered, however the Review observes from the evidence amassed on this issue that it is unlikely that many schools of nursing would adopt such a model. Much of the concern expressed about this approach centred around the perception that nursing could become diluted by the other disciplines or indeed become lost. Interestingly, while the Royal Australian College of General Practitioners were supportive of such interdisciplinary collaboration, the Australian Medical Association supported the notion of a common core in the health sciences as long as medicine was not included (National Review, 1994).

Philosophical Underpinnings

The principal aim of the new undergraduate pre-registration programmes was to provide a better professional preparation and to improve the career choices of professional nurses (National Review, 1994). The main aim of the government was to provide a flexible high quality workforce that would meet the health care needs of the Australian people into the 21st century. To these ends, a number of characteristics of the graduate were identified as ones that the programme planners should be cognisant of whilst planning their curricula. In terms of the employability of the graduates, there has been much debate in Australia about the adoption of a competency based approach to education, not just in nursing but also in a number of other areas. Such an approach advocates that the requirements of the workplace in terms of the necessary skills and knowledge needed to do the job, should be central to the learning experiences of those students being prepared for those jobs. Some have argued however that such an approach is inappropriate for a profession such as nursing in that it precludes the broader based type of education that is required to develop such attributes as critical thinking, reflection on practice, innovation and lifelong learning, to name but a few (French, 1992). In this regard, La Trobe University Faculty of Health Sciences, in its submission to the Review, suggest that many of the competency statements are expressed in simple behaviourist terms and thus

54

downplay the reflective and evolving nature of professional practice. The Faculty argues that while universities need to be mindful of core competencies in developing their curricula:

> It is not the aim of the university merely to develop a practitioner who is aware of contemporary practice patterns, but rather our graduates should be able to develop new methods of working, and evaluate proposals for new approaches to the practice of their professions. We are not aiming simply to produce automatons who can undertake mechanical tasks but rather we are aiming to graduate thinking individuals... (National Review, 1994, p. 99).

The issue of employability also involves the issue of generic skills (National Review, 1994). A number of the submissions to the Review specifically mentioned the need of the new curriculum to prepare nurses who were capable of functioning in multiple contexts, and hence the need for it to "provide a broad and sound foundation for the development of multiple skills." (p. 166). Generic skills it is felt, will enable the creation of the flexible workforce mentioned above, and includes attributes like verbal and written communication skills, analytic skills, teamwork, problem conception and solving, learning how to learn, creativity and lateral thinking. In this regard, the National Review (1994) point out that:

> University nursing schools are required to prepare students for a wide range of nursing roles and to fulfil educational goals as well as vocational goals. Graduates must be competent for registration and also prepared for other professional, intellectual and social situations that they will face. Placing nursing education in higher education serves a range of purposes, and it is necessary to hold the different elements together in a workable balance, without one purpose becoming dominant (National Review, 1994, p. 100).

These principles and attributes are the main ones that were used to guide the curriculum planners and hence, as will be seen in the section on outcomes of the programme, are those which were used to measure the success or otherwise of the programmes in the few evaluation studies that were carried out.

Programme Length

University schools of nursing in Australia are on the whole autonomous bodies and are therefore not compelled by any centralised curriculum (Marquis et al, 1993). Therefore, schools are free to determine what is taught in the curriculum and indeed there is evidence that considerable variability exists between schools of nursing (Farrell and Carr (1996). The majority of programmes are of a three year duration principally due to the restrictions that are placed by DEET (1993) with regard to financing a fourth year. However, in principle, DEET (1993) is agreeable to allowing institutions to innovate in course length and structure. (This is discussed in more detail in the section on funding).

A variety of possible variations for pre-registration degree programmes were mentioned in submissions to the National Review (1994), and these are presented in Table 2.2.

The issue of a fourth year to the pre-registration degree programme was raised in many of the submissions to the National Review (1994). Many of the arguments in favour for such an extension were built on the premise that three years was insufficient in which to fit the required theoretical and clinical instruction and hence in many cases the latter was invariably shortened. There was also the argument that all other health professionals were educated to at least a four year degree standard (National Review, 1994). Indeed, Marquis et al (1993) report that there was much disappointment among nurses when it became evident that the hard fought for bachelors degree would be less than four years in length. This disappointment was exacerbated a year later when the National Review (1994) suggested that they were "not entirely convinced" that a fourth year was justified and hence refused to recommend such a lengthening (p. 179).

TABLE 2.2. Proposed models for pre-registration nursing degree programmes

- A three year degree incorporating clinical practice.

- A three year degree incorporating clinical practice, followed by an honours year for selected students.

- A three year degree, followed by a one year internship that is preliminary to registration.

- A four year degree which spread the present undergraduate curriculum, with the expansion of certain parts, over a longer time period.

- A four year course with provision for a range of electives from non-nursing disciplines to encourage more educational breath, as some of the advocates of the transfer envisaged.

- A four year course which contains a stronger science-based stream in the first two years (this was advocated by some academics working in the science disciplines that service nursing).

- A four year course consisting of one year foundation studies in the health sciences, followed by a three year nursing degree.

- A four year course consisting of two years generalist foundation health sciences course, followed by two years nursing education with a major focus on clinical practice, entry would be common across the health sciences.

- A five year course consisting of a preliminary year of Enrolled Nurse (EN) level education to graduation as an EN, followed by three years of Registered Nurse (RN) education and a one year internship before registration (this was felt to be attractive because of the opportunity for paid employment as an EN during RN education).

- A combined degree course of perhaps five years in length, such as nursing/arts, nursing/science, nursing/business studies.

- Following an undergraduate degree in another discipline, a two year graduate nursing programme.

Source: National Review of Nurse Education in the Higher Education Sector, 1994.

Curriculum Content

Pre-registration nursing education in the higher education sector includes some subjects shared by all university schools of nursing, however, there are also wide variations in course orientation, structures and content (National Review, 1994). The Review identifies the following courses as ones which are commonly included in this programme:

- Nursing (Theory and clinical).

- Bio-physical sciences.

- Behavioural and social sciences.

- Electives.

It would also appear from the findings of a study conducted by the Review that between 50 and 80% of the programme was devoted to nursing theory and practice. Also, all courses include a substantial amount of clinical education, and all include the following basic academic subjects:

- Bio-physical sciences—   Physics; Chemistry; Biology; Microbiology; Pathophysiology; Pharmacokinetics.

- Social and Behavioural—   Sciences – Psychology; Sociology; Ethics.

The Review also identified a number of themes or strands which ran through the curricula of the various schools, including:

- Reflective practice.

- Clinical Competence.

- Lifelong learning.

- Problem solving.

- Health Service Needs.

- Multidisciplinary Orientation.

- Cultural Diversity.

French (1992) reports that many Australian educators have adopted a problem based learning approach, some for the complete course, others for specific parts of the programme. The author points to a dilemma which some advocates of this approach are confronted with, namely, how does one expose students to non-clinical related knowledge and to other disciplines if one's focus is only on knowledge pertaining to nursing practice? The author warns that if all learning is reduced to what is required for the practice of nursing, there is the risk that a narrow professional education will ensue.

Entry Requirements

The National Review (1994) reports that "cut-off scores for school leaver entry into pre-registration nursing courses are relatively low" (p. 82). It is further reported, with some concern, that a significant number of entrants into nursing did not in fact have a high preference for nursing and only entered because as low scorers on leaving school, their options were limited. Moreover, nursing in Australia is not seen as a profession of high standing (Dahl, 1992), and both intrinsic and extrinsic rewards are seen to be minimal (National Review 1994). Some expressed the expectation and indeed the hope that the move to the tertiary sector and in particular the upgrading to bachelor degree status, would have a positive effect on the quality of nurse entrants (National Review 1994).

Currently, students are required to complete a three year under-graduate degree in an approved university before being eligible to register as a nurse. Entry to university is gained by possession of a matriculation certificate after the successful completion of 12 years of schooling or the equivalent. University nursing education is available to both school leavers and to mature students. Those who wish to become enrolled nurses are required to meet less stringent criteria, namely, the successful completion of a one year hospital certificate programme in nursing (Harloe, et al., 1995).

Neill and Barclay (1989), in a study of the sociodemographic characteristics of nursing students in higher education, identify a typical student profile for students entering nursing as follows:

- Is female.

- Aged 17.

- Born in Australia.

- Speaks English only.

- Identifies with Anglo-Australian Culture.

- Gained Entry via final secondary education exam.

- Has a matriculation score between 325 and 344 out of 500.

- Has a home address in a suburb of the 10th decile- which has the highest socio-economic score.

- Has a father who is educated to baccalaureate level who is in the manager/administrator occupational group.

- Has a mother educated to high school level who is engaged in home duties.

- Attended a government secondary school.

- Does not receive AUSTUDY (Federal Government Student Assistance Allowance).

- Received information about nursing from SATAC (South Australian Tertiary Admissions Centre).

- Chose a tertiary nursing course for personal satisfaction.

2.5 Funding of Nurse Education

Health is one of the largest sectors in Australian society, employing over half a million people, and represented 8.6% of total domestic expenditure in 1991 (OECD, 1993 cited in National Review, 1994). This was slightly higher than the OECD average of 8.1% that year. As is the case in most westernised countries, the basic character of health is labour intensive, with staff costs representing about 70% of all costs. As the largest occupational group of the health labour force in Australia, nursing costs represents about half the total costs of health care (National Review, 1994).

The Funding of Higher Education

While most Australian universities are governed by State legislation, state funding of these institutions is minimal. Over 60% of the total costs of universities are provided for by the Commonwealth Government, however, in some cases, this rises to three quarters of all funding (National Review, 1994). The Review further points out that whereas both tiers of government are involved in education policy and planning, the Commonwealth is the most influential level of government, and all state/territory activities in this regard, are co-ordinated at a national level.

Funding of higher education in Australia is governed by a rolling triennium' whereby public funding is planned three years in advance, with a provision for annual negotiations over the amount of funding for the third year. The National Review (1994) points out how since 1994, the Commonwealth funding is provided in the form of a block grant for each institution (including capital grants). However, part of this cost is defrayed by the Higher Education Contributions Scheme (HECS). This scheme covers about 22.5% of average course costs (AU$ 2,500 per student) and under these arrangements, students make payments to the government which cover a portion of the public costs of providing places. HECS payments can either be paid at the point of enrolment or else can be paid through the tax system when the student enters the workforce. In some cases, students are entitled to receive means tested assistance grants. These grants can be converted to student loans and can subsequently be repaid through the tax system. While the transfer of nurse education to the tertiary sector technically made student nurses liable to HECS charges, in reality, most were exempted from these charges (National Review, 1994).

Commonwealth funding is determined by weighted student enrolments and funding per unit depends on the course of study and on whether the course is at undergraduate level or post-graduate level. Further, funding is also determined by the Relative Funding Model. This is a system which was designed to ensure that the determination of funding reflected comparative teaching costs. The model which was developed in 1990, includes a teaching and a research-related component and differentiates disciplines according to cost. Five clusters are determined by this model with law for example in cluster one and medicine in cluster five. Under this model, pre-registration nurse education is classified in cluster three, however, the model has not been applied to nursing as the initial transfer agreement quarantined nursing from the rest of higher education funding (National Review, 1994).

The Funding of Nursing in Higher Education

Transfer Arrangements

Under the terms of the Nurse Education Transfer Agreements, the States and Territories provided 75% of recurrent funding and all capital funding associated with pre-registration nurse education from 1985 to 1993. The remaining 25% was paid by the Commonwealth Government (National Review, 1994). There was however, a marked variation in the unit costs between the various states and territories. By the end of the transfer period however, this variation had been considerably reduced. Johnson, (1994) argues that it is not at all surprising that funding levels varied so much given that there were considerable variations in how States and Territories funded traditional programmes. The author cites the example of New South Wales, a State that traditionally invested well in nurse education. As a result, it was estimated that on completion of the transfer, no additional costs were incurred by this State, whereas Queensland, a State with a less generous history in this regard, estimated that the costs it would have to meet, would be considerable. Each State set its own funding level based on its own criteria and experience, and according to the National Review (1994), levels were very much determined by two main influences, namely the historic cost of hospital based training (including teaching salaries, resources, buildings etc...), and the historic cost of providing a place in the advanced education sector. This latter cost was determined by the cost of the small number of Commonwealth-funded pilot projects that existed, and also took into account such costs as equipment, capital expenditure and recurrent costs. A problem with this, according to Johnson (1994) was that there was no sound basis for some of the State and Territory estimates of historic cost, because, historically, no specific funds were set aside for nurse education. It is therefore unlikely that many of the hospitals concerned exercised sufficient controls over their nurse education budget' to enable them to make such an estimation.

The author further identifies the difficulties associated with identifying the cost of the clinical component of the traditional programme if such accounting was not adhered to, and makes the important point that this cost was often underestimated because of the student nurse contribution to hospital labour:

Few of those who were concerned with the costing of professional pre-registration nurse education in the years leading up to the transfer gave any detailed consideration to the particular costs likely to be associated with the clinical component of nurse education. Clinical activity, within the scope of hospital-based nurse education was all too often considered only as the contribution of the learners to the provision of nursing services (Johnson, 1994, p. 21).

Indeed, it was later discovered that the cost of nursing degrees was considerably more that that of generalist degrees principally due to the cost of the clinical component.

The National Review (1994) states that the funding of the move of pre-registration nurse education to the tertiary sector did not "appear to be especially generous" (p. 76). A further problem identified by the Review was that funding for nursing education that was provided by the State and Commonwealth, was not always passed on in full by the institution's finance departments. This situation was not peculiar to nursing, however, and the Review reports that despite their efforts to obtain information regarding the actual levels of funding administered to nursing in each institution, they failed to uncover much of this information as it was generally classified as "confidential" (National Review, 1994, p. 77).

That nursing was poorly positioned to bid for funds at the time of the transfer, is also an issue raised by both Johnson's (1994) discourse, and by the National Review (1994).The latter authors' cite a submission they received from the Australian Council of Deans of Nursing wherein it is argued that nurse academics, due to their large teaching commitments and their need to retain clinical credibility, are compromised when it comes to research activity and publication rates. They are therefore disadvantaged in comparison to other faculty staff who are "not required to meet the requirements of personal professional and academic involvement as well as the need to prepare students for professional registration" (National Review, 1994, p. 77). This situation prompted the Review to recommend that special research funding be made available to nursing in order to enable the discipline to establish this aspect of its academic role in the tertiary sector. The following year, Dunn (1995) paid tribute to this recommendation and the favourable response from government that followed, suggesting that such funding would indeed follow. That this funding did become available is evident from an Editorial in Collegian in 1996 wherein sixteen research projects are catalogued, the purpose of which being to address some of the issues highlighted by the National Review two years earlier.

Not all agreed however, that nursing research activity lagged so far behind as suggested by the Council of Deans of Nursing above. Indeed, Bennett (1996), whilst acknowledging that nursing's late arrival in the area has meant that the profession has had to undergo a rapid learning curve, argues that nursing's efforts in this area were being rewarded. Bennett contends that nursing research activity was indeed fulfilling its higher education academic requirements, and also, that there was much evidence of progressive nursing knowledge development as a result of these efforts. The author does express some concern however, that recent cut-backs in the funding of higher education could have dire consequences for nursing's progress in this regard (Bennett, 1996).

Post Transfer Arrangements

From 1994, the Department of Employment, Education and Training (DEET) took over responsibility for full funding of pre-registration nurse education, to a maximum of 18,980 places, at funding rates analogous to those provided by the States at the time of the transfer. Further, it was decided that there would be no equalisation of funding levels between States or institutions (DEET, 1993), this despite the recommendation of the Higher Education Council to do so (National Review, 1994). These new arrangements also meant that the Commonwealth would now fund all of pre-registration nurse education, an arrangement that was different from that for other higher education disciplines. This situation caused concern for many in the profession and prompted the Council of Deans to call for a minimum funding standard to be set. Much of the concern centred around the point that the criteria used to determine funding for nurse education was obsolete, also, the funding arrangements did not allow for research activity costs. Moreover, whilst the Relative Funding Model did not apply in the case of nursing, the post-transfer funding levels determined for nursing fell short of those specified by this model (National Review, 1994).

In 1994 the National Review stated that at present, the duration of the pre-registration course was standardised only in regard to its public funding. Schools of Nursing were free to offer courses in excess of three years in length if they wished, however, since 1995, they have had to do so at their own expense (DEET, 1993). DEET also stated that where States and Territories had funded a degree of more than three years during the transfer period, the Commonwealth would continue that funding in 1994, but would not do so after that year. Whilst insisting on this three year funding limit, DEET (1993) emphasised that institutions had complete freedom to innovate in course length and structure. Interestingly, the National Review (1994) report that the majority of Deans of Nursing were in favour of a uniform course length, the most commonly stated length being four years however. The Review further report that such an aspiration was also raised in many other submissions that they received, pointing out however, that the implications of funding this fourth year would mean an addition of $50 million of public funding per annum. Moreover, the Australian Council of Deans of Nursing (1994) argued for an eight semester degree course on the pretext that the extra time was essential to ensure that the graduates were multiskilled enough to enable them to function in any of the areas of practice that they choose to work. Similarly, the Faculty of Health Sciences at Charles Sturt university (1994) declared that no three year nursing degree was sufficient to make a beginning practitioner competent, a point with which Shorten and McMurray (1992) concur, suggesting that a three year programme was an inadequate time frame within which to provide the comprehensive education that is necessary for today's nurse. In this regard, the National Review (1994) report how clinical education was often taking place between semesters due to insufficient time within semesters, and that baccalaureate nursing education in many countries including the United States, Canada, United Kingdom, Japan, and Scandinavia, were all conducted over four years. Despite the foregoing, the Review stated that it was unconvinced that a four year degree was necessary. The committee argued that whilst acknowledging the fact that nursing knowledge and professional requirements are becoming increasingly more complex, the same might be argued for other disciplines also. The point was made that rather than increasing the length of the course, perhaps what was needed was the examination and subsequent development of such qualitative issues as clinical education, transition to work, and teaching quality (National Review, 1994).

According to Hudson (1996) the aforementioned education cutbacks in 1996 dealt a serious blow to nursing. The author reports how the University of South Australia's Salisbury Campus was set to be phased out resulting in fewer places for nursing students, and points out that rumours abound that there will be further cuts in the region of 5% to 12% to higher education, with similar consequences for nursing. It would appear that these closures are not only as a result of budget cuts, but also, that they are victim to a number of restructuring initiatives that were taking place at many universities. Hudson goes on to quote Professor Macmillan, Professor of Nursing at University of Newcastle who demands that nurses should be exempted from proposed changes in fee structures if higher education is to continue to prepare high quality professionals for the health services. Similarly, Hudson cites Olga Kanitsaki, senior lecturer at La Trobe University who argues a case for nursing students to be afforded higher fee assistance rather than cuts to same or to the introduction of higher fees. Kanitsaki makes this argument on the basis that the Government should be considerate of the fundamental inequalities that women still suffer in the workforce. Notwithstanding this, Uren (1996) argues that because nursing represents such a high proportion of the student population nationally, there is no way that nursing faculties could be treated separately from cuts to university funding (cited in Hudson, 1996).

Funding the Clinical Component

Attempts at quantifying the cost of the clinical component of pre-registration nurse education are fraught with difficulty (National Review, 1994). The review recounts how in the traditional hospital based programmes, hospital budgets simply accounted for the contribution of student nurses to hospital staffing, after deductions of their wages. A study in 1978 by Bennet and Wallace found that for the major hospital based courses, the cost was one-sixth that of nursing courses in advanced education. This difference was chiefly as a result of salaries and other academic costs, however, it would appear that the cost of the clinical education component was not a specific factor in these calculations. Little changed when it came to estimating the cost of the clinical component for the new programme. Johnson (1994) points out that:

> Very little attention was paid to the idea that clinical experience, planned and implemented to achieve educational objectives rather than the needs implicit in nursing service delivery, might be a significant source of pre-registration nursing education costs. Clinical teaching/learning, as distinct from workforce participation, was not identified as a component of the educational programs of hospital-based student nurses; consequently, it was not costed (Johnson, 1994, p. 52).

Johnson argued that the historical situation whereby students were a cheap part of the workforce, and whereby staff often engaged in clinical education out of goodwill rather than on the basis of some form of contract, became the precedence by which the costings for that component of the new course were determined. Hence, the author asserts, nursing commenced the transfer to the tertiary sector on the assumption that clinical education costs needed little specific attention (Johnson, 1994). This was not the case for all of the Australian States and Territories however. The National Review (1994) report that the New South Wales Health Department had indeed carried out the required costings of the new programme in this regard, and also had come to formal arrangements with a host of prospective clinical placement education sites. These agreements set out the respective rights and obligations of both parties namely, the university and the health agency.

In 1993 Brennan, noted that patient dependency and staffing systems did not always accommodate the weighting that should be applied to areas providing clinical education. The author also indicates how recent health reforms that resulted in changed budgetary practices and methods of resource allocation, rarely took into account the clinical cost of professional education for students other than medical students. Brennan also draws attention to the fact that in some areas staffing levels have been so low that managers have had to withdraw placement opportunities in the interests of both client and student safety (Brennan, 1993). Furthermore in this regard, Johnson (1994) suggests that the combination of financial cut-backs and the obligation placed on clinical staff to provide clinical education for the new breed of student nurse, (who is no longer a part of the workforce, and whose qualifications will be superior to their own), has frequently lead to a situation of growing intra-professional intolerance. Bennett, (1996) expresses concern that such financial pressures could lead to a reduction in the number of undergraduate nursing students (and hence staff), and also could result in a reduction in the clinical component of the course. The author acknowledges that the cost of the undergraduate programme is high in comparison to other degree programme, principally as a result of the strong clinical component that exists. Bennett argues that clinical competence is impossible to achieve without quality experience in the clinical areas, therefore, "any attempts to reduce further the expensive clinical component of our programmes must be resisted strongly. (p.3). In a similar manner, Madjar, (1995) argues that clinical placements, during which students can relate with actual clients and work alongside expert registered nurses is a vital constituent of the pre-registration programme. Despite this, the author argues, nursing departments are severely under-resourced to provide optimum learning experiences for their students. Whilst acknowledging that nursing degree programmes are costly, Madjar points out that such programmes have brought large numbers of students (and hence revenue) into universities, therefore, the author argues, universities need to be committed to providing adequate resources so that they can be taught well (Madjar, 1995). Indeed the National Review (1994) report that the majority of submissions from schools of nursing and many of the student nurses who were surveyed expressed concern at the lack of clinical placement sites, a lack of variety of placements, and also a lack of quality placements. Moreover, the Royal College of Nursing of Australia noted that there was widespread dissatisfaction with the arrangements for undergraduate clinical education, calling for an appropriately weighted funding plan in which the costs of clinical education were sufficiently explicated (National Review, 1994).

Kaur and Gallagher (1995), the former a mature nursing degree student, point out how nursing students are increasingly faced with difficulties both in accessing accommodation whilst on their placements, as well as in meeting the associated costs of these placements. The authors point out how the degree course at James Cook University, North Queensland, requires fulfilment of 950 clinical hours during the three years of the programme. Students are constantly faced with the ongoing costs associated with clinical placements the authors argue, which include travel ($100), accommodation ($150 per week), food ($100 per week), extras ($50 per week), double rent ($100 per week) and loss of income ($100). This can mean that each placement costs the student in the region of $700-$800, which over three years could amount to $4,800. One consequence of this expense is that prospective nursing students seek alternative courses of study. Kaur and Gallagher (1995) conclude that there is the risk that students who cannot afford these expenses are disadvantaged and further, as a consequence, nursing could become an elite profession, commenting that: " It would be a tragedy if students who are motivated to stay in this profession leave because of financial difficulties" (p. 17).

Indeed, one year earlier, the National Review (1994) had anticipated such hardships for students, particularly those working in remote rural areas, and as a result, they recommended that supplemental funding be made available to offset this situation.

However, at least one senior nurse respondent to the Review suggested that student nurses should pay for these placements. Moreover, in general the Review commented that:

> it is likely that the resources available for clinical education are deteriorating and that the total level of funding may need to be increased. It is also clear... that the funding of clinical education eds to be stabilised. (National Review, 1994, p. 211).

The Review further emphasised that the matter should not be allowed to drift, and that a clear line of responsibility needed to be established whatever the source of funding. The Review further expressed the opinion that it was not reasonable to expect the higher education institutions to assume the full costs of the withdrawal of State funding.

A number of authors, including the National Review (1994) have made suggestions as to how further revenue could be generated, or as to how costs could be shifted. For example, Bennett (1996) suggests that all post graduate courses should be fee-paying, and further asserts that nurse educators need to become much more entrepreneurial, pointing out that the possibility of paid consultancies and the generation of income from abroad needs to be explored in depth. The National Review (1994) however proposed that if a portion of the pre-registration student weighting were transferred to post-registration courses, the numbers of undergraduate students requiring clinical education would fall thus enabling some improvement in the resourcing of clinical education within the same total expenditure. Regarding the funding of preceptor training, the Director of the Nursing Branch of the South Australian Health Commission expressed the view that funding for all clinical supervision of this nature should come from the education budget and not from health. Similarly, a submission to the Review from Queen Elizabeth Hospital in South Australia complained that the costs of teaching and supervising students in the clinical areas, plus the costs of educating new graduates to a competent level in the graduate nurse programmes, were unfair, particularly as it was felt that new graduates were not adequately prepared for their clinical role and hence did not represent value for money (National Review, 1994).

Funding Graduate Nursing Programmes

The National Review (1994) observes that financing of the Graduate Nurse Programs (GNP) is generally acknowledged as being a health sector responsibility. The cost of these programmes is normally met directly from the budgets of the hospitals and other health agencies involved, the main costs being those for nurse educators for the programme (often part-time /casual), administration, as well as the wage costs of the participants. Generally, participants to these programmes are supernumerary for the theoretical part of the programme but not during clinical placements. Other costs concern those associated with preceptor arrangements, primarily in regard to the re-distribution of their workloads for the duration of the course. The Review also points out that in some cases in the private sector, participants in the GNPs contributed themselves to the cost of the programme. In this regard the Review cites a comment by one of the organisations that forwarded a submission to the committee, the Australian Hospital Association:

> In private hospitals in South Australia, graduate nurses pay $1000 for a competency-based program which assist their integration into nursing. They are happy to do so since it provides guaranteed employment and a supportive entry into nursing. Pay deductions are available on demand....The raising of this type of fee is not yet common practice in private hospitals in other States (National Review, 1994, p. 230).

This situation the Review believes is likely to develop further, given the role of GNPs as a potential gateway to employment (National Review, 1994).

In Victoria, it is reported that the Department of Health and Community Services (DHCS) funds GNPs at the level of half of a first year staff nurse salary. The funding is available to all acute hospitals and therefore small rural hospitals are able to become involved thus ensuring them a small but constant supply of new graduates. Without such a scheme, clearly these hospitals would be unable to fund such programmes.

2.6   The Changing Role of Nurse Educators

The transition to university and bachelor degree status brought with it major changes to nurse education and consequently, there were considerable implications for nurse educators in terms of role, work priorities, and conditions of employment. Essentially the transfer meant that the hospital-based schools of nursing either closed or redirected their focus towards post-registration education, in-service training and Graduate Nurse Programmes (National Review, 1994). In its submission to the National Review, the Department of Employment, Education and Training commented:

> DEET has the expectation that, with the completion of the nurse transfer agreement, or soon thereafter, all faculties of nursing will be indistinguishable from other academic faculties: within the nursing discipline the full array of academic activities needs to be pursued, including scholarship, research within the discipline and multidisciplinary research (DEET, 1994, cited in The National Review, 1994, p.325).

This was indeed a tall order for a profession new to academia, and in the following sections, some of the implications of this expectation will be outlined.

A Change in Culture

One of the major implications of the transition for nurse educators was that the cultural environment was different, if not alien to some (National Review, 1994; French, 1992). Nursing education found itself in a new system of management with different procedures for financial accountability, administration and course accreditation. The National Review (1994), whilst acknowledging that there was much evidence that the quality of nurse teaching often surpassed that of the tertiary sector, there were too many instances of a pedagogical approach to nurse education, with didactic teaching methods being used and resource intensive high contact hours. In the universities, greater emphasis was placed on advanced education and on such academic activities as research, presentations, and publications, which are time consuming on the part of the educator.

The high emphasis on teaching is common in nursing French (1992) argues, however, this does not fit well with the academic model of higher education where teaching is seen as only one of the academic's many roles. French further asserts that in many instances, nurse educators transfer their concern for the welfare of patients to promoting the interests of their students. Their time therefore, becomes consumed with teaching and other student related activities often to the detriment of their own career development (French, 1992). Moreover, nurse educators soon discovered that the amount of support that they received from the university, and their capacity to control resources, were to some extent dependent on their ability to secure research grants, something they were unaccustomed to doing in their previous places of employment (National Review 1994;

Marquis et al, 1993; French, 1992). They were also confronted with the prospect of having to secure overseas marketing, commercial research, consultancies and fee-based post-graduate education (National Review, 1994), this despite the fact that many staff lacked the training and expertise to take on such roles, at least until some time after the transition was complete (National Review, 1994; French, 1992). A number of factors complicated this situation, including the fact that many nurse educators were at the time of the transition busily engaged in course development, university-based teaching, and in some cases clinical practice (National Review, 1994), while other problems arose as a result of the hurried implementation of the new programme in some centres, and many educators were at the same time pursuing further studies at advanced degree level (Madjar, 1995).

According to French (1992), the move from the traditional nurse education programmes to the university system, required a major paradigm shift on the part of nurse educators. In particular the author argues, adopting the academic culture requires nurse educators to reconcile two potentially conflicting roles, namely those of nurse and academic. French cites Sutton (1991) in this regard, who suggests that:

> [nurse educators] enter the higher education sector shaped by their experiences as nurses .... the result of which is the development of attitudes, values, beliefs and behaviours which make their adjustment to the academic role particularly troublesome (Sutton, 1991, p. 1).

French (1992) argues that nurses are socialised in such a way that a service orientation is integrated into their very persona, and that this is expressed as a desire to help others and to be caring. Conversely the author argues, the professional socialisation of university academics is one of integrating a scholarly orientation into the persona of an individual whose choice of an academic career is generally the expression of a desire to advance knowledge through teaching and research. This situation may lead to the professional-academic dichotomy which is described by Mauksch and Styles (1982) as a conflict between values: service versus scholarship and accountability versus detachment. When nurses become academics therefore, they must incorporate two incongruous roles (French, 1992). The service role behoves that time and concern be devoted to the well-being of others, while the academic role requires the investigation of the internal and external universe, dealing with abstractions and having little knowledge of or caring how the quality of life of others is improved through one's actions. Success in this latter role French argues is very much dependent upon a selfish approach to work whereby the academic must protect time for scholarly activity. That nurse educators had few if any role models to emulate when considering whether or not to transfer to university faculties is evident from a comment made by Townsend in 1991. The author is cited at length here in order to give the reader a full appreciation of the dilemma that faced many nurse educators:

> In 1984 nurse education in NSW was propelled forcefully from the hospital based apprenticeship training system to the tertiary based studentship education system. Nurse educator were caught in a dilemma. At the extremes there were hospital loyalists who saw it as treason to desert the existing system and the college breakaways who saw the opportunity of a lifetime. Between these there was the majority group who perceived merit in both situations. They were torn between supporting a system which had served them well but which was diminishing and maintaining their careers by adopting the new system, the realities of which were not yet known to them. In the end, over the first few years several hundred nurse educators applied for academic positions in colleges across NSW. For most it was a leap into the unknown. There were few role models or mentors. There were no existing faculties into which individuals could quietly slip and maintain a low profile until they found their way (Townsend, 1991,p. 69).

In addition, Moorehouse (1992) points out how many nurse educators accepted academic positions without having much knowledge of the expectations and norms of the academic setting. Further, the author argues, very few had had the privilege of being a full-time university student themselves. It is perhaps not surprising therefore that certain authors have suggested that nursing has been accorded only a token acceptance in some universities (Crowther, 1994; Marquis et al., 1993; French, 1992). Moreover, Mason (1991a) suggests that at the outset, nurse educators were unfamiliar with the power sources within the university setting and often did not understand the rules, the author adds however that this situation is rapidly changing with nursing faculty quickly becoming politically astute.

The Need to Upgrade Qualifications

The aforementioned Sax Report (1978), in anticipation of the imminent changes in nurse education, recommended that nurse educators should be prepared in "selected institutions which have expertise in the education of adults,..[and that] those with capacity' were encouraged to take 'advanced courses.' " (p. 118-120). Similarly, the Noble Report (1974, cited in Russell, 1988) suggested that the success of future nurse education programmes was primarily dependent upon the adequate supply of nurse teachers. The committee therefore stressed the urgent need to increase the number of nurse teachers as well as to develop the current teacher resources. Despite these recommendations, evidence is that there were not enough suitably qualified nurse educators to participate in this cultural revolution (National Review, 1994; French, 1992). One professor of nursing told the National Review in 1994 that:

> At the time of the transfer, there were insufficient numbers of suitably qualified nurse educators to develop the new programmes; some schools chose to recruit scholars from North America, New Zealand and the United Kingdom to meet this shortfall. The strain on nursing faculty was, nevertheless, considerable... (National Review, 1994, p.78).

Nurse educators had requested access to advanced educational degrees for many years prior to the transfer according to Marquis et al (1993), however, many obstacles stood in their path the authors claim. One result of this is that a two-tiered system, similar to that obtaining in North America began to develop in Australia (French ,1992). In this system, research and other academic activity is reserved for those academics who have doctoral level preparation, leaving the less academically qualified educators to conduct most of the teaching and other service activities, especially at undergraduate level. The result of this system is the development of an elite cadre of educators, this at the expense of the development of other faculty staff and of educational research programmes. Lowery (1991) warns of further implications of this system. The author describes two types of academic, the "superstar" and the "putting out to pasture." The former is where a "superstar researcher is engaged to carry out a project thus necessitating a substantial amount of the faculties resources to be given to that individual. All too often, the author asserts, the superstar's energies are directed towards her/his own interests rather than those of the research potential of other staff. The purpose of engaging the superstar is not to develop the team, rather it is to bring prestige through her/his academic achievements. The "putting out to pasture" on the other hand is where those faculty members who are deemed to have least research/academic potential are given more teaching loads and other service commitments, in particular at undergraduate level (Lowery, 1991).

When the move to the tertiary sector began, many states were caught short of having adequate numbers of educators with advanced degrees (Marquis et al, 1993). As a result, pressure was placed on nursing faculties in the universities to facilitate nurse educators to attain such degrees, the result being that during the early stages of the transfer, many nurse educators were busy pursuing their own studies. Similarly, Madjar (1995) points out that at the time of the transfer, the lead-time was too short and the resources that were necessary to prepare nurse educators for their new positions were often not yet in place, hence the majority of educators found themselves in the unenviable position of having to complete their own graduate studies while at the same time engage in curriculum development and carry a heavy teaching load. As a consequence, many nurse educators came near to work related burnout (National Review, 1994; Marquis et al., 1993).

Such was the need for nurse educators to acquire advanced degrees, the National Review (1994) recommended that a special programme dedicated to staff development in nursing be established for a limited period of about five years. The Review further states that such a programme should aim to ensure that 70% of nursing academics hold higher degrees and 30% hold PhDs. The Review cites findings from the Centre for the Study of Higher Education survey (CSHE, 1994, cited in National Review, 1994) that in 1993, 44.3% of nurse educators surveyed had higher degrees and only 7% had PhDs. The Reviews proposal would bring nursing into line with other academic disciplines in terms of their qualifications, however, it is acknowledged that in the natural and social sciences, a higher proportion than 30% hold PhD degrees (National Review, 1994). The review further recommends that one of the criteria for awarding grants should be the development and maintenance of active links with health agencies and professional bodies in the health sector in order to strengthen the relationship between professional practice and academic research. Moreover, French (1992) offers some suggestions as to how academic departments could assist in the development of nurse educators, regardless of their academic achievements. The author suggests that orientation programmes should be developed to help the new academic adjust to their role and the culture of academia, that mentorship programmes be set up whereby established scholars are utilised for their expertise in scholarly activity, that workshops on grantsmanship, publication and teaching be established, and that annual career development sessions be conducted with all academic staff (French, 1992).

Increase in Workload

The National Review (1994) report that respondents in one of their surveys were almost evenly divided between those who felt that the workload of nurse educators had increased and those who felt it had not. Some were of the opinion that workloads were increased due to a reduction in resources while some felt there was a decrease primarily due to a decrease in student numbers and/or a reduction in student contact hours. The latter was not necessarily due to reduced resources however, many reporting that the transition in some schools from high contact teaching to more moderate methods had resulted in a decrease in workload (National Review, 1994). Perhaps the most commonly mentioned contributory factors to a perceived increase in workload were those discussed earlier in this discourse, namely the pressure to attain higher degrees and to engage in other scholarly activity, as well as the short lead-in time to the transition. Indeed, Mason (1991a) suggests that many were unable to keep up with all these pressures and either succumbed or struggled on with the scholarship requirements and the politics of academe.

The Need to Develop the Research Role

One of the natural consequences of the transition to the higher education sector was the need to develop research in nursing (National Review, 1994). Research is an activity that is formally required in all universities and increasingly, the level of funding and other forms of support for non-research activities are dependent on the success in competitive research grants. The Review proposes three reasons why it is important to develop a strong higher degree/research profile. These are:

- The need to develop nursing research itself;

- Research and innovation provide favourable conditions for all branches of academic endeavour;

- Research training and higher degrees enable academics to teach and supervise post-graduate students.

Whilst acknowledging that many nurse academics are committed to research activity, the Review observes that even if current trends in enrolments for PhDs and masters degrees continues, the numbers of nurse academics with PhDs would still fall short of one in three. Moreover, the majority of those who hold masters degrees in nursing did not pursue masters studies through research only. Indeed, Madjar (1995) argues that Australia's nursing research culture is only beginning to emerge and is very much limited by the lack of research degrees in nursing. Hence the author points out, many nurses pursue research degrees in other disciplines. This is further evidenced by Harvey's (1988) account of the experiences of a nursing graduate whereby the author on the one hand praises her nurse teachers for instilling a good research appreciation in students, but on the other hand recounts the frustration experienced by her peers and herself when trying to locate up-to-date Australian Nursing Research when completing assignments.

The pressure of work particularly the urgency to attain higher degrees has also been implicated as a factor contributing to poor research development in nursing by Marquis and colleagues (1993), while the National Review (1994) illuminates the difficulties encountered by prospective nurse researchers in trying to secure funding for research.

A number of initiatives have been developed to try and further advance nursing research. For example, La Trobe University has set out to double PhDs among nurse academics and in other centres, honours streams in bachelors degree programmes have been established (National Review, 1994).

Notwithstanding the foregoing, Marquis et al., (1993) contend that there is evidence emerging that Australian nursing is developing its own body of knowledge and hence becoming less dependent on American and British research. The author cites Lawlor's research on somology (how nurses manage the bodies of others) and Townsend's development of the interaction-oriented healthcare facilitator model of self-care, as examples of such developments.

2.7 Clinical Learning

The purpose of clinical education in nursing is to enable the student to exercise the previously acquired knowledge to patient care situations and to attain the kinds of professional and personal skills, attitudes and values thought essential for entering the health system (Wong and Wong, 1987). In the pre-registration nurse education course in

Australia, theoretical and clinical components of the programme are integrated so as to enable the nurse graduate to attain the level of clinical competence that is necessary to engage in professional nursing practice (National Review, 1994). Clinical education was the most commonly cited issue of all of those raised in submissions to the National Review, (1994), thus bearing testimony as to how important this aspect of nurse preparation was seen by those concerned. The National Review (1994) also points out that there was much evidence from the submissions received by the Review that there was "considerable anxiety about clinical education" among members of the profession (p. 185).

Length of Clinical Placements in the Under-graduate Degree

In 1992, the Australian Council of Deans of Health Sciences carried out a survey of the faculties of health science then in existence (N= 23), achieving a 100% response rate. A number of academic disciplines including nursing were included in this survey and it is reported that approximately two thirds of all nursing programmes participated. The findings of this survey suggest that the average amount of hours devoted to clinical practice in pre-registration programmes was 894 (range 508-1226) (ACDHS, 1992 cited in National Review, 1994).

In 1994, the National Review as part of its terms of reference conducted its own survey of clinical education in nursing in Australia. The findings of this survey demonstrate that the total hours of clinical education in the under-graduate degree ranged from 354 to 1770 hours over the duration of the programme. Most schools it was found provided approximately 600 hours and in over half of those schools surveyed, more than one third of the total course time was devoted to clinical education. Furthermore, only a modest amount of clinical education was provided in the first year of the programme, this gradually increasing as the programme progressed. The Review suggests that the amount and type of clinical education provided was very much dependent on the registration requirements of the State and Territory concerned, and by the educational programme of the school of nursing and the resources available to it. This latter point is important as it will be seen later, that many of the problems with clinical education came about as a result of a lack of adequate resources. The requirements of the various States and Territories in regard to the amount of clinical education that is necessary for registration as a nurse varies considerably. Some States specify a minimum number of hours and/or a minimum range of clinical placements. For instance, the Victorian Nursing Council require a range of from 900 to 1000 hours while the Queensland Nursing Council specifies a minimum of 900 hours (National Review, 1994).. Interestingly, the aforementioned survey conducted by the Review would seem to suggest that few schools were meeting these requirements, however, it is not clear from which Council's jurisdiction these schools come.

With regard to the format, number and duration of clinical placements, the National Review (1994) identified the following from its survey on clinical education. Three main forms of clinical experience were identified:

- Block placement for several continuous days at a time, on a recurring basis, over a period of several weeks.

- Weekly placement for one or two days a week throughout a semester.

- A combination of these two, e.g.: weekly placements in year one and two, block placements in year three.

It was also found that the length of time in placement per day varied. Some students undertook a complete eight hour shift while others worked for one or two hours at a time, depending on the arrangements of the school. Those programmes which were longer than three years normally provided an extended period of clinical placements in the latter part of the programme (National Review, 1994).

Regarding the format of clinical placements, the Royal College of Nursing, Australia (RCNA) in its submission to the Review commented:

> The trend in nursing education, to expose the student to as many clinical settings as possible, usually for a relatively short period of time, is not necessarily the most useful. The student gets a "taste" of many different areas of nursing but runs the risk of developing very little confidence in any. For the beginning practitioner, which is the outcome of all pre-registration programs, it may be more productive to provide a smaller range of placements for any one student but allow more time to develop confidence and skills (National Review, 1994, p.200).

Interestingly, research conducted by Battersby and Hemmings (1991) suggests that the quality of the clinical educational experience may be more important than the quantity. The researchers studied a cohort of nurse graduates who were working in five different public hospitals in Sydney. Clinical experience was operationally defined as on-site clinical education such as that taking place in hospitals, nursing homes and community health centres, but not laboratory work or clinical simulations. In the study, students' clinical performance was rated independently by the researchers and by nurse managers and the performance of those rated as "low clinical group" was compared with that of "high clinical group". The researchers discovered that those who had fewer hours of clinical experience ("low clinical group") seemed to differ little in their clinical competence from those who had more hours of experience. The National Review comments on this research pointing out that the findings did not prove that there was no positive relationship between the hours spent in clinical education and student competence. The Review further suggests that it is possible that the results were affected by a variation in the quality of the different programmes. Also, the Australian Nursing Council Inc., (ANCI) (1993) commented in this regard that whilst it is recognised that the quality of the clinical experience is of greater significance than the quantity, it stands to reason that "there would be a minimum quantity of clinical experience (whatever this might be) below which it would not be possible to obtain quality" (p. 197). Moreover, Johnson (1994) suggests that the findings of Battersby and Hemmings (1991) were used to argue against extending the degree to four years, something that was advocated by many on the grounds that three years was not enough time to fit in the required theoretical and clinical instruction.

Venues for Clinical Placements in the Under-graduate Degree

The aforementioned ACDHS (1992) survey identifies public health institutions as the most common location (84% of clinical education in nursing) for conducting clinical placements for pre-registration nursing students. The National Review's (1994) survey is more explicit on such locations however, reporting that all schools of nursing surveyed conducted clinical placements in acute care hospitals, and all except one in community settings. Furthermore, over 50% of schools provided placements in mental health, paediatric or elderly care settings while over 30% provided such placements in developmental disability, community mental health, or extended care. There is also evidence of a shift of emphasis from hospital to community settings, as advocated by the World Health Organisation's (1985) Targets for Health for All by the Year 2000.

Notwithstanding the Reviews finding that over 50% of students are provided with a clinical placement in mental health care settings, Farrell and Carr (1996) found that the amount of time that students are exposed to theory and practice of mental health nursing varies considerably from school to school. The researchers conducted a survey of all schools of nursing in Australia requesting information on the mental health aspects of their curricula. There was an 84% response rate and the authors report how in one school of nursing, undergraduate students had 30 hours of mental health theory and no practice while another had 128 hours of theory and 200 hours of practice. When one considers that in Australia, pre-registration degrees are now generalist and graduates can practice in any of the disciplines of general nursing, psychiatric nursing or paediatric nursing, these findings imply that students could graduate and enter practice as a mental health nurse with little or no theoretical and/or clinical experience of the discipline.

Moreover, there is also evidence that in some situations schools had difficulty in accessing sufficient suitable clinical placements for their students. For instance, the National Review (1994) report that certain schools of nursing were finding it difficult to provide clinical placements to students especially in mental health care, this primarily due to the fact that there was a reduction in the number of hospital beds as a result of the restructuring of the health services. Similarly, the Australian Nursing Council (ANCI) (1993) reported that the greater throughput of patients and the trend to greater acuity in hospitals, and in particular the de-institutionalisation of mental health care, meant that there was a reduction in the availability of clinical experiences for student nurses. The result of all of this was that there was competition between schools for scarce clinical placement opportunities. Shortages were most severe in paediatrics and mental health which for States like New South Wales was particularly problematic given that students in this State are required to fulfil placements in these areas.

Resourcing of Clinical Education

There has been some debate in the literature as to who should resource the clinical educational component of the pre-registration nurse education course. The Department of Employment Education and Training (DEET), in its submission to the National Review (1994) rejects any possibility of the higher education sector having to fund and resource this part of the programme. DEET insists that the clinical component should be "industry-funded" and that the situation that pertains with regard to clinical education, whereby the Health sectors of the respective States and Territories resource clinical education, should remain. The Department also rules out any additional funding in this regard, in its submission. Conversely, the Department of Human Services and Health (HSH) expresses the view that the cost of any shift of clinical contact teaching to the health system should be accomplished within the existing education budget, rather than it being an supplementary cost to the health sector. This is not to suggest that the higher education sector should carry the full cost of clinical education, rather, that any increase in clinical education over the levels applying during the transition period should be covered by education (National Review, 1994).

Clinical education is resoursed on a large scale. For example, the National Review (1994) report that at the Curtin university of Technology, 45% of academic staff time and 50% of all resources are vested in the clinical component of the programme. Further, in

1993, it is reported that this university spent $3 million in clinical supervision alone. Similarly, the ACDHS (1992) suggest that the cost of clinical education is huge citing the example of New South Wales where the hourly rate for part-time clinical supervisors was $28. A typical nursing programme in this State with 200 students and 900 hours of clinical work therefore faced a potential annual bill of $680,000, including clinical teaching, travel and other costs. Further, this body points out that there was little prospect of additional public funding for this component of the course as a result of tightening public health budgets. (Problems with the clinical component of the course due to funding anomalies have already been discussed).

Teaching and Supervising the Clinical Component

Clinical placements generally occur in off-campus health service settings such as hospitals and occasionally in clinical skills laboratories on campus. Nurse educators and registered nurses both participate jointly in the clinical programme.

The National Review (1994) identifies a number of personnel who are engaged in and share responsibility for clinical education of pre-registration nursing students:

- University academics who were RNs currently registered to practice, and teaching both theoretical and clinical aspects of the programme.

- University academics from another discipline, often paired with a nursing academic.

- University academics who specialised as clinical teachers and taught only in the clinical part of the programme.

- Jointly appointed clinical teachers who were employed by both the university and the health care agency.

- Practitioners from the health care agency where the students were placed, employed by the health agency but seconded to the university for the duration of the programme.

- RNs from the agency where the students were placed, appointed to act as preceptors.

- RNs from the agency where the students were placed, who might be working alongside the students and whose teaching role was informal and probably unacknowledged.

- Sessional clinical teachers who were not attached permanently to either the university or the health care agency and who specialised in clinical teaching. These sessional teachers were usually selected by the university and not the health agency.

Essentially there were three broad groups of clinical teachers: academics in the university schools of nursing, the sessional teachers and the staff from the health agency. Different selection procedures, role preparation, payment, and relationships with the higher education institution pertained for each group (National Review, 1994). Further, the Review reports that the majority of schools of nursing surveyed expressed the view that the ideal minimum qualification for the clinical teaching role was a Registered Nurse certificate and a bachelors degree. Moreover, all rated clinical competence higher that academic qualifications for this role. With regard to the role of clinical teachers, the National Review (1994) provide a summary based on one of it's submissions, of the various activities that academics working as clinical teachers were required to perform. These include management of laboratory sessions, formal lecturing in the classroom, preparatory tutorials in advance of clinical placements, debriefing sessions- sometimes on a daily basis during clinical placements, teaching by example and role modelling, preparation for specific programmes of clinical education, clinical supervision in community settings, and the conduct of in-service classes to orient hospital staff.

Cawley, et al., (1994) observe that the models of clinical teaching used by the universities range from the traditional model in which full responsibility for students' clinical teaching is taken by faculty, to a model in which this responsibility is shared with hospital staff nurses who are formally appointed as clinical teaching associates. In a model used by Monash university, and reported by Grant, et al., (1996), clinical teachers are either nurses employed by the university on a sessional basis or are nurses working in health care organisations who are relieved of their clinical responsibilities and seconded to, and paid by, the university to supervise and teach students during their clinical placements.

In the survey of schools of nursing that was undertaking by the National Review (1994), it emerged that in the majority of schools, between 50 and 100% of nurse academics engaged in regular clinical teaching. Indeed, it is further reported that in seven of these schools, all academic staff engaged in this area of teaching. It also emerged that there was a general expectation in all of the schools surveyed that academic staff would keep up to date in their clinical skills, the most common way of doing this was seen to be through clinical teaching. Schools were also of the opinion that not alone would clinical teaching accord staff some level of academic credibility, but also, that it was a valuable way of establishing and maintaining networks with the clinical areas. The Review further reports from this survey however, that there were significant numbers of clinical staff who did not engage in clinical teaching, the most common reason cited being high workloads and consequent lack of time.

The above survey also found that sessional staff or health agency staff were employed for clinical teaching in about half of those schools surveyed. These staff were cheaper to employ than academic staff for the universities and it was also possible to deploy them in a flexible manner, for example in small blocks of time as needed. The Review further notes that while many of these staff were deemed to be high quality teachers, some were felt to lack adequate teaching preparation and others had weak attachments both to the academic programme and to the health agency. That clinical teachers lacked adequate preparation is also finding of Hart and Rotem's (1994) study. This survey, based on interviews with 30 final year nursing students, found that while students felt that it was important to have a supervisor who was knowledgeable of the clinical setting of the placement, having a supervisor who was not a member of the university teaching staff and who was not au fait with the curriculum might be a disadvantage. Dunn (1995) agrees with this view and with the recommendations of the National Review in this regard and emphasises the need for clinical facilitators or preceptors to be clinically credible and to have current expertise in the specialist area in which the students are having their clinical placements. The author further argues that these personnel must be familiar with and maintain a strong link with the theoretical component of the curriculum, and must also have an indept appreciation of the clinical objectives that are set out for students. One way of doing this the author argues, is to integrate the clinical experts with the educational specialists, working in tandem towards mutual goals (Dunn, 1995).

Moreover, in a study conducted by Grant, et al., (1996) of the attitudes of clinical nurses (n = 304) towards their teaching role with university nursing students during clinical placements, the authors found that most staff (97%) saw this as part of their role. Further, they felt adequately prepared to undertake this role (79%) and gained much satisfaction from it. Of concern however was that less than half (46%) felt that students were adequately taught by the nominated university clinical teacher. When asked what information and expectations they had about the course and the universities role, their responses concur with those of Dunn (1995) above. Staff wanted to know about students level of education and about the universities expectations of students during their clinical placements. Further, they expected university clinical teachers to be accessible and to be involved with teaching their students clinical aspects of practice. The survey of clinical teaching conducted by the National Review (1994) discovered that while approximately 50% of all schools of nursing ran some form of preceptorship/clinical supervision education programme. only one quarter provided provided academic staff and sessional teachers with such a facility. The Review further reports that some nurse academics who were teaching in clinical programmes lacked up-to-date practice, similarly, some nurses from clinical areas were not familiar with the nature and requirements of the course. In this regard, a submission by St Vincent's Hospital to the Review stated:

> The quality of supervision and clinical teaching also causes great concern. Much of the supervision is provided by educationally unqualified and clinically inexperienced nurses employed by the universities. While espousing the value of clinical teaching, employment of junior or agency staff to provide this vital element of the student's experience demonstrates the tertiary sector's lack of commitment (National Review, 1994, p. 201).

That many schools of nursing provided clinical preceptors for their students is also evident from the National Review (1994). For example, a survey conducted by the Private Hospitals' Association in 1992 demonstrated that 80% of students on clinical placements in their hospitals had a clinical supervisor. Sixty per cent of these were provided by the university, the other 40% by the hospital. However, it is also evident that there were problems in this regard, not all hospitals were offering this level of supervision. Further, it can be argued that all students should be offered this service. Due to the increased use of medical technology and the greater acuity of patients, most students were deemed to require intensive clinical supervision, however, in many instances staffing constraints and tight budgeting of resources in general made this level of supervision problematic. Moreover, there is also evidence that some students were used as part of the workforce whilst on clinical placements principally due to low staffing levels. The National Review cites a submission from the Australian Nursing Federation in this regard:

> ...It is well recognised that many agencies reduce the number of staff or alter their rostering arrangements when students are out on clinical placements and providing patient care. This is not only an underhanded cost shifting exercise, but also severely hampers the possibility of educative supervision and thus changes the student's placement from an educative experience to a pair of hands role (National Review, 1994, p.199).

Further, the average student to supervisor of 10:1 was deemed to be too high and limited the effectiveness of the clinical programme. This was also evident from Grant et al's (1996) study, the authors suggesting 8:1 as the generally cited ratio. In reality, the authors point out, the ratio is frequently higher than this with one clinical teacher likely to be responsible for students placed in many areas of a large hospital or on different campuses of the same hospital. As clinical teachers are unable to provide adequate supervision, some universities place a heavy reliance on the pairing of registered nurses working in clinical areas with students who are providing hands-on care (Grant et al., 1996). In this survey, respondents expressed the view that they expected clinical teachers to be accessible to their students, however, concern was expressed at the amount of supervision required of individuals as evidenced by the comment: "There are too many students for the clinical teacher...{and clinical teachers] ...need to be on the ward more often than they usually are,... I realise however, this person cannot be everywhere at one time" (Grant et al, 1996, p. 28). Similarly, Robertson (1993) reports that over 30% of student nurses surveyed suggested that they had insufficient contact with clinical teachers from the university, as well as with academic staff and part-time sessional staff. In this regard, Wong and Wong (1987) argue that academic staff in higher education often do not value highly clinical teaching primarily as it is not accorded the same prestige as other academic pursuits.

Because of these types of situations, the Executive Director of Nursing Services at Woden Valley Hospital, Australian Capital Territory, in a submission to the National Review (1994) called for adequate provision for the funding of sufficient numbers of clinical supervisors for undergraduate students, and also for funding for the release of clinically based preceptors to supervise students. Indeed, Bennett (1996) warns that there is a risk that attempts will be made to reduce the clinical component of the programme due to the associated high costs.

With regard to the funding of clinical supervisors/preceptors, the aforementioned Private Hospitals' Association survey (1992) point out that 90% of hospital based supervisors received extra payments, working on average 9.6 weeks per year in this capacity. The authors suggest that as clinical education benefits both parties, in principal hospitals are happy to fund such ventures. In practice however, many are finding it difficult to do so for financial reasons. It also emerged from this survey that "some hospitals found that they were getting more requests for placement and have to consider either allocating more staff or refusing requests" (p. 3).

A separate survey by the Australian Private Hospitals' Association Limited in that same year(1992), found that 81% of their member hospitals accepted pre-registration students for clinical placements. Almost 65% of these hospitals used their own qualified nursing staff as preceptors and over half paid their preceptors for this work in addition to their normal salary.

2.8   Outcomes of the Pre-registration Undergraduate Programme

The transfer of registered nurse basic education to the university sector has resulted in a decisive change in the nursing profession in Australia (French, 1992). Not only has nursing taken its place alongside the other professions, but the prevailing expectation is the development of a different kind of nurse because the new nursing programmes represent a stronger commitment to encouraging students to develop critical thinking abilities and on applying these abilities to clinical practice (National Review, 1994). This section will consider to what extent these ambitions have been realised.

Employers Perceptions of Pre-registration Programme and its Graduates

In 1994, the National Review reported on a survey which it had commissioned (Robertson, 1993) that sought the perceptions of employers, academics and nursing students of the pre-registration under-graduate nursing programmes. In this study, 1,102 employing institutions out of a total of 3,000 were surveyed, however, the response rate was poor at 26%. This figure rose to 59% for hospitals with 200 beds or more. Employers were instructed to rate the pre-registration programmes on a scale of one to five, according to a number of criteria. The results of this rating are presented in Table 2.3.

TABLE 2.3. Employers' perceptions of the pre-registration programme

Criterion	Rating
The criteria that were rated the highest were:	
• Responsiveness to community needs and trends	3.4
• Responsiveness to changing technologies and procedures in health care	3.4
• Preparation of graduates to meet community care needs	3.2
Lowest scoring criteria were:	
• Articulation of courses with education programmes for Assistants in Nursing (AINs)	2.0
• Articulation of courses with education programmes for Enrolled Nurses(ENs)	2.4
• Transition of graduates into health care workforce	2.6
• Preparation of graduates to meet acute hospital needs	2.6
• Responsiveness to employers advice on curriculum development and implementation	2.6

Source: National Review of Nurse education in the Higher Education Sector, 1994.

TABLE 2.4. Strengths, weaknesses and proposed modifications to the programme

Characteristic of Pre-registration undergraduate programme	Proportion of Employers naming this characteristic
	%
Strengths	
Broad theoretical base	77
Attitudes to profession	32
Interpersonal skills	25
Attitude to learning	21
Range of experience	19
Intellectual skills	19
Personal characteristics	16
Separation of education and service	13
Weaknesses	
Lack of clinical competence	77
Time management/organisational skills	39
Inadequate preparation for employment	33
Inadequate clinical exposure	22
Programme content	13
Theory to practice problems	12
Suggested Modifications	
More clinical and practical experience	72
Improve transfer to workforce	36
Increase health-education liaison	26
More reality focus	21
Better planning of placements	14
Hospital based preceptors	10

Source: National Review of Nurse education in the Higher Education Sector, 1994.

Employers were further asked to identify the strengths, weaknesses and possible modifications of these programmes. From these responses it became evident that the greatest concern related to the clinical competence of graduates, while their greatest strength was seen to lie in their broad theoretical base. There was also a strong focus on graduates immediate transition to professional practice, and on the hands-on skills of the new graduates. What became most evident from the overall responses of employers was that there needed to be better liaison between health and education sectors in programme planning, and this was mentioned explicitly by over one quarter of all those surveyed (Robertson, 1993). Table 2.4 lists the suggested strengths, weaknesses and issues for modification that were common to ten or more per cent of respondents.

Employers were then asked to rate the graduates on a five point scale with regard to a number of attributes. The results of this rating are presented in Table 2.5.

TABLE 2.5.   Employers rating of nurse graduate attributes

Attribute	Rating
Those that rated strongest were:	
• Motivation to continue own professional development	4.0
• Verbal communication skills	3.8
• Written communication skills	3.7
• Appropriate professional values	3.6
• An appreciation of the role of research in developing nursing practice	3.6
• An understanding of major bio-ethical issues in health	3.6
• Ability to work in multidisciplinary teams	3.4
• Ability to apply natural and social scientific theories to nursing practice	3.4
Those characteristics which rated weakest were:	
• Ability to prioritise work	2.5
• Ability to manage the delivery of care to a group of clients/patients	2.7
• Technical skills in nursing	2.8
• Understanding of the policies, politics and funding of the health care system	2.8
• Understanding of the factors affecting future health care provision	2.8
• Basic nursing skills	3.0
• Ability to respond to different health care needs	3.0

Source: National Review of Nurse education in the Higher Education Sector, 1994.

It is important but not surprising to note that, after one year of nursing practice, graduates demonstrated a great improvement in their ability to prioritise work, to manage the delivery of care to a group of patients, and in technical skills. For example, ratings for practical skills rose after one year from 2.9 to 3.7, communication skills from 3.7 to 4.0, while skills related to understanding increased from 2.9 to 3.4 (Robertson, 1993).

In conclusion, the researcher points out that graduates faired poorest in their hospital-related skills, function better in community settings, and have a good grasp of some aspects of the context of health care, but not so of its organisation. Further, it was noted that they possessed good interpersonal skills. Also, graduates strong orientation to their own professional development was seen as indicating that the concept of lifelong learning that was central to many of these programmes, had taken hold (Robertson, 1993).

Students and academics in Robertson's survey were reported to have rated the new graduates higher than had the employers, the main differences were noted in ratings of practical skills. This discrepancy the researcher contends may be due to the different focus and goals of these groups of individuals, but of more concern, may also mean that academics expectations of the graduates were too low, that they are out of touch with the requirements of the workplace, or that they were unaware of the actual standards (or lack of) that the graduates had actually achieved (Robertson, 1993).

Other Outcome Studies

There is a paucity of research on the outcomes of the pre-registration undergraduate programmes in Australia and this is not only an observation of this writer, but is also a view that is supported by the National Review (1994).One such study, reported on in some detail, is that by Happell (1996). In this study, the researcher examined the perceptions of registered psychiatric nurses of the differences between tertiary (university) and hospital based nursing graduates. A comparative study was conducted between two groups of psychiatric nursing students, one group who received their nursing education in the university (n = 25), the other who received their nursing education in a hospital based school of nursing (n = 20). All students were interviewed in depth during the third year of their course and again on completion of their first post-qualifying year. The researcher points out that the information gleaned from these preliminary interviews was supported by data from further interviews conducted with five educators of the hospital based course, nine from the university course, and four registered psychiatric nurses who had acted in a supervisory capacity for the subjects. The data from the above preliminary interviews was then analysed and clustered to provide categories for the main study interviews. In the main study, four registered psychiatric nurses (2 supervisors from graduate nurse programmes, one clinical nurse specialist and one director of nursing) were interviewed during which information was sought on the following issues:

- Discernible differences detected between the two groups in terms of clinical competence, theoretical knowledge and attitudes and approach to their work.

- The manner in which university based graduates had adapted themselves to their role as registered psychiatric nurses.

- The manner in which university based graduates were received by other staff in the hospital.

- Whether any distinguishing characteristics of the university graduates had been sustained during the period of employment and/or were considered to be sustained in the future.

- Positive contributions if any, that the university graduates have made to psychiatric nursing as a profession.

- Perceived strengths and weaknesses of the two courses gained as a result of the experience of employing tertiary based graduates and hospital based graduates.

All of those interviewed suggested that the university educated students were less clinically competent and less confident than students from the traditional programme a view also expressed by employers in Robertson's (1993) study. Clinical skills were perceived to be less developed in the university student group, a situation that was seen to cause considerable anxiety for these nurses. One such comment was:

> ...There's often a gap or lack where they try to bring their practical skills up to mesh in with their theoretical skills...due to lack of opportunity to practice. Whereas hospital people tended to have more hands on practice... (Happell, 1996, p. 114).

Notwithstanding this, it was felt that the university educated nurses did not take long to attain a level of clinical competence at least equal to that of the traditionally educated nurses. Many registered nurses employed in the study hospitals, it was reported, expressed concerns about the university students prior to the employment of the first cohort, these however, were quickly dissipated once they experienced the university graduate nurses at work.

As a result of their broader education, university students in this study were seen to have a wider view of psychiatric care than their traditional student counterparts. They were also seen to be more flexible, more enthusiastic, highly motivated, and to have a broader perspective on patient care. Happell (1996) cites a number of other studies (D'Cruz and Bottorff, 1986; McCue, 1982; Dowdall, 1979; Brooker, 1978) which suggest that the traditional training was narrow and restricted in focus, the author suggesting that data from the present study seems to indicate that this deficiency is being redressed by the new programmes. As a result of the perceived greater flexibility, the university graduates were considered to be less entrenched in the existing system, and therefore more able to reflect upon it, as evidenced from the following quote: "...I think they're probably less accepting of the system they work in ...They tend to be more reflective about what they are doing, rather than just coming in and doing it and bitching about it and going home..." (Happell, 1996, p.115). Respondents also expressed the view that unlike the traditional students who felt once qualified that was it, they knew enough about nursing to get on with the job, the university graduates were more likely to recognise their own needs in terms of ongoing education. Moreover, the depth of theoretical knowledge demonstrated by the university educated nurses was seen by respondents to promote a desire for learning among other registered nurses. This concurs with the findings of a small study at the University of Sydney Faculty of Nursing whereby it was found that the attitude of traditionally prepared RNs had changes towards further education, this as a result of them experiencing the new graduate nurses in the workplace. This study, reported in the National Review (1994), indicated how there was a pronounced increase in interest in further studies in the traditional RN population and the demand for places in conversion courses was so great that it outweighed the number of government places that were available. The main disadvantage of the university programme that respondents in Happell's study cited was that these nurses spent too little time in the clinical areas. However, this was considered to be a short term problem that was quickly overcome after graduation.

While these findings must be considered with some caution primarily due to the nature of the study and the small number of respondents, the findings are presented in some detail here due to the fact that there are so few studies of this nature. Further, the results are important as they concur somewhat with those of Robertson (1993), and with some of the UK outcome studies cited in chapter one.

Pelletier, et al., (1994) surveyed the effects of graduate nurse education on clinical practice and career paths of a convenience sample of forty registered nurses (RN). While the present discourse concerns undergraduate pre-registration programmes, this study is included here as it is felt that it may illuminate some outcomes that are in common with these latter programmes. In this pilot study, a forty three item questionnaire was administered to 40 RNs in the final week of their course of study. Respondents were asked to identify any personal effects of graduate studies that they perceived. An increase in self-esteem, assertiveness and confidence were among the main facets identified (52.5%), with feelings of satisfaction, fulfilment and being challenged also mentioned (12.5%). Some adverse effects such as stress, limits to social life and pressure of time were also identified (30%). Respondents were further asked about any changes in professional thinking that they felt had come about as a result of their present studies (see Table 2.6). As can be seen in this Table, over 40% identified cognitive effects such as questioning, reflection and improved insight into practice, while feelings of self-confidence and satisfaction in their work were also suggested. There were also perceived benefits to their professional relationships and to their professional standing (Pelletier et al, 1994).

The researchers also report that 52% of the group planned further studies in nursing with only 7% not interested in this. The remainder were undecided in this regard. Of those who intended to pursue further studies, most identified a masters degree in nursing as their choice of course. Such an appreciation of the need for further continuing education was also evident from the findings of Robertson (1993), as reported earlier.

TABLE 2.6.   Changes in professional thinking during graduate studies (n=40)

Changes	Number	%
Cognitive effects on practice: — questions and thinks about practice. — insight into nursing and health care. — improved decision making. — increased knowledge and application. — need for continuing education.	16	40
Feelings about work: — self-confidence. — esteem. — positive. — satisfying. — improved job prospects.	13	33
Relationships: — respect for co-workers. — improved communication with professionals. — increased professional standing.	8	20
Did not respond:	3	7
Total	40	100

Source: **Pelletier et al., 1994.**

The National Review (1994) report that a large proportion of the submissions that they received from the profession centred around the issue of whether or not the transition of nurse education to the university sector had in fact achieved its objectives. The overwhelming majority of these submissions believed that it had and that the transfer had established a new culture of professional education for nursing. The Review reports on a number of local studies that were carried out to see what positive outcomes had come about as a result of the new programmes. One such study at Flinders University School of Nursing, compared it's first five cohorts of graduates with their predecessors from traditional programmes. The results suggest that the graduates had a stronger orientation to career advancement than the hospital trained RNs. The findings of the study further indicate how the numbers of graduate nurses applying for further study or seeking positions as nurse academics, clinical teachers or holding positions on various professional or academic committees, was far greater than those from the traditional group.

Despite all of these perceived benefits from graduate studies in nursing, the National Review (1994) point out that these changes have not necessarily translated into a significant increase in upward job mobility in nursing. While the effects of the transition to university based education have on the whole been positive, the Review argues that an expansion of effective career opportunities depends on more than just educational reform. It also depends on the level of resources available in the health agencies, the employment market for registered nurses, and the situation regarding promotional and managerial positions. That some university graduates were unable to find work after graduation, is also identified by the National Review (1994). As a result, some of these graduates emigrated, while others chose different career paths and hence were lost to the profession.

Transition to work

Graduate transition concerns the passage from higher education to the workplace. It is the period of learning and adjustment to the requirements of professional nursing practice during which the graduate acquires the skills, knowledge and values required to become an effective member of the nursing workforce (National Review, 1994).
Difficulties in transition to work are evident in many occupations and are not peculiar to nursing. Such difficulties are most prevalent when the educational programme has been full-time and the most commonly cited are reality shock and periods of low work productivity on the part of the graduate. Difficulties particular to nursing often relate to feelings of fear and anxiety at the prospect of having to cope with emergency situations.

In order to ease this transition period, the Australian Nursing Council Incorporated (among others) state that following registration there should be a period of transition before the newly graduated nurse is expected to function as an autonomous member of the nursing workforce:

> Pre-registration nursing courses are designed to prepare a beginning practitioner to provide safe, competent and responsible nursing care in a variety of health care settings...registering authorities expect that on initial registration, a beginning practitioner will have access to more experienced nurses. Registering authorities would not expect the beginning practitioner to take in-charge positions or function alone in areas where clinical decisions involve unpredictable outcomes or where the patient client presents with multiple problems (National Review, 1994, p.215).

In particular, it has been observed that new nursing graduates are lacking in clinical skills and confidence (Happell, 1966; National Review, 1994; Robertson, 1993), however, Ives and Rowley (1990) suggest that this perception may be exacerbated by the fact that graduate nurses are often shown antagonism by traditionally prepared RNs. While experienced nurses might be expected to display some empathy for new recruits undergoing the same educational programme that they did, graduate nurses are seen as being quite different, with more education but less practical experience than their predecessors. Therefore, the attitude of some traditionally prepared RNs was found to be one of ambivalence towards them. Ives and Rowley (1990) argue that the attitude of RNs to university education was very much a function of where they trained. In their study 87% of graduate nurse managers were favourably disposed towards graduate preparation for nurses, and felt that the profession stood to benefit from this situation, only 27% of non-graduate nurse managers agreed with this view.

A number of models have been proposed as ones that may assist in the transition to clinical nursing practice including:

- Graduate Nurse Programmes (GNPs).

- Short Orientation Programmes.

- Preceptorships, Mentorships, Buddy systems etc....

- Internships.

Graduate Nurse Programmes

Graduate Nurse Programmes (GNPs) provide a broad milieu in which activities such as orientation schedules, preceptorships and other forms of support may be provided. They vary in length from about six weeks to just over one year, and in some cases are considered a preliminary to an offer of employment (National Review, 1994). Two main types of GNPs were identified from the various investigations carried out by the National Review namely, the deficiency model and the skills consolidation model. As the name suggests, the deficiency model is grounded in the assumption that the new graduate is lacking in some respects and therefore, the GNPs role is primarily to correct this deficit. The consolidation model on the other hand is built on the premise that the graduate needs a period of supervised practice in order to strengthen clinical and decision-making skills, and to orientate her/him to the workplace and to the professional culture. Further, the role of GNPs varies between the States and Territories (National Review, 1994).

In the survey of employers conducted by the National Review (discussed above), in excess of 90% of respondents felt that such programmes were necessary, while almost 60% of those surveyed offered these programmes in a range of health care settings. The National Review (1994) gives an example of a typical GNP pointing out that these programmes usually include an initial orientation or induction schedule, some theory classes, and a system of preceptored clinical practice. It would appear that the theory component of the GNP is usually small, the Review suggesting a theory to practice ratio of 1 to 28. One problem with the GNPs is that not everyone was able to gain access to one. The National Review reports that only 75% of graduates were able to gain access to these programmes. The funding of GNPs has already been discussed (National Review, 1994).

Internships

An alternative method of managing the transition process is that of a period of internship. This usually takes the form of a period of comprehensive clinical practice analogous to that of a medical internship. Under this paradigm, graduates might receive no registration or interim registration as a nurse until the graduation stage at the end of the period of internship (National review, 1994). The main aim of the internship is to give students an opportunity to consolidate their clinical skills and knowledge of the job.

The debate on a four year degree also drew attention to the possibility of an internship. This option represented to some an attractive solution to the problem of facilitating the development of the skills component of the job in a programme that was heavy with theoretical content. An internship year would allow a large portion of clinical practice to be compacted into one year, and would also extend the time available for other parts of the curriculum (National Review, 1994). In effect, the Review argues, this would mean a four year course (3 years plus 1 year internship). A major concern with the development of internships and four year nursing degrees is the associated costs. An intern year in a pre-registration programme would mean that student nurses therefore need to be paid a proportion of a graduate nurses salary, and also, because it would be necessary to provide internships in a variety of settings, with travel costs for those who must journey to remote areas.

Notwithstanding the financial implications of an internship at the end of the undergraduate programme, a number of other issues were debated. The Australian Nursing Council Inc., (ANCI) (1993) pointed out that one of the most important goals of nurse education is to integrate theory and practice, hence it is argued, a clinical component is not just something that is tacked on at the end of the programme. The Incorporation argue that approaches such as GNPs, internships, and provisional registration are remedial in response to the perceived deficiencies in the clinical component of the course. It was also foreseen that there would be problems with the implementation of an intern year, particularly in terms of what to include in such a year. It is unlikely that all graduates would have the same needs and require the same amount and type of remediation. ANCI further questions how the quality of such programmes would be regulated, and further expresses the concern that an intern year could be merely regarded as a source of cheap labour for hospitals. In effect ANCI states, an argument for an intern year is the same as an argument for a fourth year and that this latter issue should be pursued further (ANCI, 1993).

In its final report, the National Review (1994) failed to endorse the case for an internship, principally due to the belief that this approach was deemed likely to widen the theory practice gap in nurse education. Not surprisingly, the financial implications of an intern year was also seen as prohibitive not least because nursing is such a large profession, but also because it was felt that some nurses would not be able to attain a place on an intern programme and hence future employment prospects could be jeopardised. In this regard, the National review recommended:

> The Committee believes that the clinical competence of new graduates can be guaranteed without resort to internships or any other system of delayed registration. The proposals for a compulsory extended clinical placement and a joint health-education assessment of clinical competence will be a less expensive and simpler way to address the issue and one which will build the relationships necessary for the transition from university to work, rather than create new potential conflicts (National Review, 1994, p. 242).

Madjar (1995) calls for this situation to be resolved pointing out that it is not reasonable to expect nurse educators to prepare students for a university degree as well as registration as a generalist nurse in the same time that it took to prepare nurses for one specialised programme to certificate or diploma level in the past. The author acknowledges the many calls for an intern year as a solution for this problem, however, suggests that Australia should have learned from the American and Canadian experience and held out for a four year degree. In 1996, an editorial in Collegian, the Royal College of Nursing, Australia journal, gave details of a study being commissioned by the Minister for Employment, Education and Training to further consider this issue. The project, entitled Transition from Education to Employment: From University Student to registered Nurse, is designed to elicit essential planning information, which will ensure that the transition from university student to graduate nurse in the workforce is managed efficiently and cost-effectively. The editorial goes on to point out how evidence to date from the undergraduate programmes suggests that the new graduate is not fully utilising education-based skills and knowledge and perhaps more worrying, is often not attaining job satisfaction. It would also appear that many employers are providing what are described as "expensive and often inappropriate year-long de facto 'internships' (graduate nurse programmes) for new graduates, which [have] developed over the years based on little, if any, research" (p.11). The project, which will extend over an eighteen month period, will it is hoped provide the necessary data with which to develop a new model of student-to-RN transition (Collegian, 1996). Clearly this issue has not been resolved and as can be seen from the foregoing, many hospitals continue to give de facto internships (and in some cases full four year degrees) either at their own expense, or else at the expense of the student.

2.9   Changes in Nurse Education – New Zealand

The Move to the Higher Education Sector

According to Williams (1992), the first efforts to move nursing education to the higher education sector in New Zealand occurred as early as 1912. While the author does not elaborate on the nature or format of these early efforts, she does suggest that the propelling force behind this ambition was the belief that in order for nursing education to develop, it needed to be moved from a service setting to an educational setting.

In 1971, a review of nursing education in New Zealand was undertaken by Dr Helen Carpenter. The main recommendation of this review was that comprehensive programmes of nurse education based in the tertiary sector should be established, and that hospital-based programmes should cease (National Review, 1994). Dr Carpenters transfer proposal was soon after accepted by the Government and in 1973 a new system for the educational preparation of nurses in New Zealand was introduced. The move from the apprenticeship style hospital based system to three year diploma nursing courses within the general tertiary education system began. A further change in Government policy towards nursing education came about in 1978. In that year, the Government stated that its goal was now to move nursing education completely into the tertiary education system (Horsburgh, 1989). Horsburgh states that a phased programme of transfer had taken place whereby as the number of new students ("comprehensive students") increased, the number of traditional students decreased. Furthermore, the service contribution of the traditional students had been taken over by extra qualified staff, and since 1988, Horsburgh asserts that most nursing care was delivered at that time by qualified nurses.

Sherrard (1995) reports that up until the Education Amendment Act was passed in 1990, both nursing and midwifery education was offered at diploma level in the polytechnical colleges. The author points out however, that within the education sector there has been considerable disagreement about the significance of the academic qualification "diploma." Moreover, Sherrard comments that "these programmes have all now become bachelor degrees in either nursing or health science (nursing)" (p.2). This move from diploma to degree status did not however mean a move from the polytechnics. These colleges continue to provide pre-registration nurse education, however, now at degree level. Indeed there has been much debate on this issue of pre-registration nursing degrees, and for a long time it would appear that little consensus had been reached. For example, Watson and Young (1994) quote at length the recommendations in this regard of the Review of the Department of Nursing Studies at Victoria University of Wellington:

> It is obvious to all that the profession of nursing is in major transition: it is in the process of growing up and emerging as a health profession and academic discipline in its own right. During this interim time of difficulty, we believe it is necessary for the profession to make a hard transition into an academic model that prepares career professionals and provides a continuum of education from polytechnic degrees to graduate research and advanced practice and teaching opportunities. ... we are convinced that due to current circumstances and all the concomitant problems and changes in nursing, women in society, and health care, the real need of nursing education within the next decade and beyond is to prepare nurses through graduate education (Watson and Young, 1990, p.19. cited in Watson, 1994, p.3).

Horsburgh (1990/91) argues that there is no doubt as to whether or not nurses should be prepared to degree level. New Zealand nurses have fought long and hard for degrees the author says however, she laments the fact that there is reluctance in some quarters to follow the world-wide trend of baccalaureate preparation for all nurses. Horsburg further comments that never has there been such a need for highly qualified nurses for New Zealand's health service. Leaders for nurses are needed as are critically thinking, creative and broad minded nurses. Such nurses the author believes will undertake the research that is necessary in order to develop nursing's knowledge base. Horsburgh also comments on the fact that other vocational and health professional groups are educated to degree level, yet there seems to be an expectation that nurses must tread a long and arduous path before they are granted access to degrees at pre-registration level (Horsburgh, 1990/91).

In 1996, there were 15 polytechnical colleges offering pre-registration nursing courses (O'Connor, 1996, Sherrard, 1995), and between them, they offer pre-registration nurse education to approximately 5000 student nurses (Gallagher, 1995). Horsburgh (1989) suggests that the overall objective of the transfer was to produce nurses who could render an improved standard of nursing care within the changing health service. The tertiary education sector it was believed, could offer nursing a broad knowledge base by integrating the biological and social sciences into nursing studies while maintaining a focus on community health as well as on the care of the hospitalised sick. However, in 1996, Wilson warns that due to changes in the funding arrangements for students' clinical education (discussed below), there is now a risk of destroying these curricular efforts at integration, and of re-introducing the theory practice gap. As a result, the author calls for the re-opening of an old debate, that of the proposal to integrate nurse education into the universities. This proposal first became an issue in 1973, as it was the only recommendation of the Carpenter Report to be dropped.

Furner (1996) supports such a move. The author accuses the polytechs for mistreating nursing students and nurse education in general. Furner claims that polytechs are immoral in that they hold on to students who are clearly not academically able for the nursing programme, until such time that it is safe to drop them from the programme. By this she means that the polys will not fail students until the last date by which they can recoup their fees, has passed. Until that date, it is alleged that these students will be kept on by the skin of their teeth through the use of action plans and learning contracts, this in order to boost their grades. As a result of this, Furner supports the call for university based preregistration education for nurses, primarily as she feels that universities are more democratic and hence are more likely to be fair to students (Furner, 1996). Not all nurses are in favour of a move to the universities at this point in time however. For example, Jill White, Professor of Nursing and Midwifery at Victoria University warns that such a move is premature. The author is cited in O'Connor (1996) as follows:

> There is an enormous danger that, in moving in that direction too quickly, nursing education would be subsumed into medical schools. Nursing education clearly needs to stay separate until it is more mature in its post-graduate studies and research base (O'Connor, 1996, p. 29).

Financing of Nurse Education

Pre-registration under-graduate nursing students in New Zealand according to Gallagher (1995), have to pay their own fees and they receive little other financial support. In 1996, Wilson reports that currently course fees are around NZL$3000 per year. As a result of this the author asserts, most students engage in part-time employment to support themselves through the programme. Wilson (1996) comments that while it is difficult to be exactly sure of how much the Ministry of Education pays the Polytechnics for preregistration nursing students, it is understood to be in the region of NZL$10,000 per equivalent full-time nursing student per year. Wilson further points out that some "market-driven" polytechs have recently increase student fees, this as a result of new financial arrangements concerning student nurses clinical education. Polytechs are now also negotiating contracts with health care providers for access to their clinical areas for student placements. While the government expects this to result in a more efficient delivery of nurses clinical education (as such negotiations are believed to create a competitive environment), the reality of the situation according to Wilson is that hard pressed students are going to be further compromised financially. Indeed Gallagher reports in 1995 that health budget holders are now calculating the cost of student supervision by clinical nurses. Currently this cost is passed on to the polytechs, however, Gallagher warns that the polytechs may soon pass this cost on to students' course fees.

The issue of student hardship is also discussed by Stodart (1990/91). The author suggests that these are hard times for student nurses. Financing their nurse education is a constant struggle and for many there are no jobs on graduation. Indeed it would appear that in some cases only 50% of new graduates have secured employment within a year of graduation (Williams, 1992). This situation according to Stodart (1990/91) pertains as a result of restricted nursing budgets, the result of which is that not alone is it impossible for new graduates to get experience, but also it is difficult for them to pay off the debts that have accumulated over their three years' studentship. Wilson (1996) comments that the main reason for conferring full student status on student nurses was to reduce the stress of combining their studies and their service commitment. The author argues that in fact the opposite has occurred. Students are being used as a source of cheap labour while they acquire clinical skills, and lack of financial support means that many have to work part-time. This is further compounded by the fact that many have family responsibilities. Wilson comments in this regard:

At least when they trained in hospitals they were paid albeit a pittance, for the service they provided, and accommodation was available at a reasonable cost. Now student nurses in the second and third year of their course are expected to work eight-hour shifts to obtain their clinical experience in hospitals (Wilson, 1996, p.27).

In return for this free labour there is not so much as a free meal provided as a token of appreciation by the health authorities, who are clearly exploiting student nurses (Wilson, 1996).

O'Connor (1996) lays the claim that there is a risk of nursing education becoming elitist due to the high costs incurred by the student. The author cites a paper presented by Barbara Wilson, National Director of the New Zealand Nurses Organisation (NZNO) whereby the author argues that one consequence of this elitism is that nursing will not be able to attract the range of applicants needed to provide an appropriate and accessible health service. O'Connor in conclusion asserts that there needs to be a more unified approach to the public funding of health allocation, both in terms of the amount allocated and also how it should be allocated. "Funding needs to be looked at in a more comprehensive way. We need to look at how public funding can be applied within and across disciplines for the future", the author comments (O'Connor. 1996, p. 29).

One final issue in funding to be reported here is that raised by Wilson (1996) regarding the manner in which the polytechs manage the nursing course funding. This the author argues is not all spent on nursing education. Rather, these monies are redistributed in the name of equity to finance new courses and to subsidise those courses that cannot be self-supporting. In this regard, Wilson claims that nursing education could be seen as what in management jargon is termed a "cash cow" (p. 27). This term the author points out was coined to refer to a well-established company with a large market share and slow growth, providing a replenishible supply of cash to be milked off to nourish the hungry newborn, (Wilson, 1996).

Polytechs have done very well out of nursing education Wilson (1996) argues, most of them having experienced tremendous growth over the past 20 years. With 5000 pre-registration undergraduate nursing students bringing with them government funding to the tune of NZL$10,000 per year per student for three years means that nurse education has become a multimillion dollar industry for the polys. With nursing courses polys are assured of their income for three years so therefore they can project their budgets accordingly (Wilson, 1996).

Transition to Work

An undesirable aspect of the undergraduate nursing programme is that some graduates experience difficulties in the transition from the student role to the staff nurse role in their first staff nurse positions (Taylor et al., 1981). Indeed there is both anecdotal and research evidence to suggest that there were in fact such difficulties (Prebble and McDonald, 1997; Stodart, 1990/91; Horsburgh, 1989). For example, Stodart (1990/91) argues that one of the reasons why there is so much graduate unemployment is that employers do not want to hire new graduates as they are perceived to be less productive initially than their experienced nurse counterparts. Furthermore, the Chief Nurse Adviser in New Zealand commented in this regard that:

There has been anecdotal evidence of some employer dissatisfaction with newly graduated nurses. Employers maintain that new graduates are not able to 'hit the decks running' and prefer to employ experienced nurses as they provide more value for money. It is interesting to note that many employers do not appear to view orientation of newly graduated nurses as an employer responsibility (Gillian Grew, Chief Nursing Adviser, New Zealand, cited in National review, 1994, p. 217).

Horsburgh (1989) conducted a study of graduate nurses' adjustment to initial employment using a natural field work methodology. This is an ethnographical approach whereby the researcher participated in the first three to four months of the new graduates employment in general hospital settings. The subjects in the study were 10 graduates from one school of nursing who had successfully completed a three year course and registered as comprehensive nurses in New Zealand. The author points out that the characteristics of the subjects were the same as other graduate groups in terms of age, gender, and previous nursing experience. A number of data collection approaches were adopted including questionnaires, participant observation and field notes. Indeed most of the data were generated from the field notes. Horsburgh found that the reality of nursing practice experienced was very different from what they expected. While the curriculum emphasised patient centred care, the experience was a task oriented approach. It was observed however, that the new graduates did possess the necessary skills and knowledge to function in the workplace notwithstanding the fact that this required them to compromise the values of nursing education. In particular, graduates were frustrated and experienced much conflict as a result of the overwhelming emphasis on the physical and technological aspects of patient care. There was a paucity of planned continuity of patient care and little opportunity to follow through the outcome of their nursing care. Overall it was felt that adjustment meant the acceptance of nursing as a system of managing certain tasks. Graduates did not resist this situation as they felt powerless to do so and as a result most expressed job dissatisfaction and many expressed guilt.

The predominant model of transition to work that was identified in this study was that of apprenticeship whereby, emphasis was placed on how to function in the workplace rather than on the refinement of clinical skills. It is also reported in this study that during their initial employment, nurses experienced some confusion regarding their role as registered nurses. On the one hand all of them received negative feedback about their clinical and work performance, however, this the researcher suggests contrasted with their nursing education where great emphasis had been placed on the development of clinical skills with clear standards and where frequent feedback on clinical performance was given. It also transpired that there was no delineation between work that was appropriate for a new graduate and that for a more experienced RN. The demands of the situation dictated how the responsibilities were apportioned, and frequently new graduates were given sole responsibility, on evening shifts predominantly, for a large group of patients. This contrasted very much with the situation on the morning shift where nurses were encouraged to adopt a role of dependence on senior nurses. There was also a perceived lack of opportunity to develop autonomous independent practice, hence, new graduates struggled to identify what was expected of them and to practice as competent registered nurses.

Horsburgh (1989) observed that graduates seemed to have difficulty in coping with unexpected or unplanned events, and that they were slow to recognise their responsibilities for supervision of enrolled nurses and students, and in the administration of medicines. Horsburgh (1989) also contends that the rhetoric and reality of the school of nursing is different from that of nursing practice experienced by new graduates. Furthermore, major conflicts and frustrations result from these discrepancies in values and practice. The researcher suggests that in the end, graduates come to accept the reality of nursing as a series of tasks, however, this is not without its costs. It is somewhat disappointing when one considers that many hopes were vested in these new comprehensive graduate nurses, in particular, the expectation that they would become key change agents. Horsburgh further expresses the hope that this may yet materialise when a critical mass of these nurses are in clinical practice.

The argument was also made that some of these nurses' experiences may perhaps be attributed to the fact that ward management practices in New Zealand at the time of this study, were substantially the same as those which pertained in the 1960s and 1970s. This means that junior staff nurses function very much as apprentices just as they did over a decade ago. In conclusion, Horsburgh (1989) comments:

> Nursing education cannot continue to educate nurses for a system of practice that is likely to lead to alienation in the first few months of employment. It is essential for nurse educators to work co-operatively with the administrators, managers and clinicians within hospitals to clarify the nature of desirable nursing practice. (Horsburgh, 1989, p. 616).

In 1997, Prebble and McDonald conducted a qualitative descriptive study of the lived experience of comprehensive nurse graduates (n=4) in their efforts to adapt to nursing in a mental health setting. Interviews were conducted with subjects focusing on current work experiences and on how the philosophical beliefs and values derived from their educational preparation fit with those encountered in the practice setting. The participants were employed in acute wards and had worked there for between six and eighteen months. Three of them were female, one male and all had been selected using a snowball sampling technique.

Three main themes emerged from the findings namely:

- Passage of transition into practice,

- Conflict,

- Contradiction.

The most frequently cited category was the Passage of Transition to Practice. All participants commented on the process that they either had or were experiencing in transition to the RN role. Four sub-themes were identified:

Lack of Orientation and Formal Support

The length of orientation periods for nurses ranged from none to a brief period, for example, one day. This mainly comprised of details concerning hospital administrative procedures as opposed to nursing procedures. Participants stated that what they needed was guidance and feedback on how to deal with specific nursing situations. However, they stated that they received very little feedback of this nature or on their performance, nor were they provided with a preceptor.

Reliance in Self

Participants spoke of having to assert themselves in order to be given any orientation, in-service education, or any other type of support needed for safe practice. They had to depend very much on themselves to gain skills and to access supervision and in-service education.

Support from Colleagues – All but one of the participants commented on the support given by colleagues. Interestingly, much of this support came from other comprehensive graduates.

The Process of the Nurse in Transition

During the interviews, the new graduates described a situation of moving from what they saw as a position of vulnerability whereby graduates limited their practice in order to remain safe. One such comment was:

> ...I also avoided...to respond to alarms. I knew that some people had to respond to alarms and other people had to stay behind to look after the ward because I was concerned that I would run there and wouldn't know what to do (Prebble and McDonald, 1997, p. 33).

The researchers however, report that these students became more assertive within six to twelve months of graduation, yet they still felt that they were taking some risks in their practice.

The second theme that was identified in this study was that of conflict. All respondents mentioned conflicts regarding the different philosophies within wards. Much of this conflict related to the fact that the students were educationally prepared to practice from an holistic perspective. However, the medical model was the predominant philosophy of the wards. One student complained:

> Yes its very medically orientated, not like a social system at all, its medically orientated and I have found that when I have tried to put a nursing perspective on someone's care and treatment, it's been removed and I have been told by a couple of people that it's not a good idea to do that, because that's not what the ward likes (Prebble and McDonald, 1997, p. 33).

The final theme was that of contradiction. All four graduates mentioned contradictions in philosophies of practice. Many of the nurses were seen to be operating from different philosophical perspectives and this often lead to friction between staff. Contradictions were also evident in students own practice. One student described how when there were many disturbed clients on the ward she had to deviate from her normal mode of practice and become more of a disciplinarian. While all of the participants in this study felt that they were adequately prepared for basic nursing in mental health settings, they did not feel prepared for dealing with what they termed specialised disorders or for dealing with complex situations or behaviours.

While a major limitation to this study is the fact that there were only four participants, all of them expressed similar views on the issues raised. Moreover, some of the themes identified here are similar to those of Horsburgh (1989) despite the fact that eight years separate the two studies, and also, they were focused on different disciplines of nursing. It is also of note that similar difficulties in transition to practice are evident from the findings of studies in other countries. Prebble and McDonald, (1997) also draw attention to the fact that a number of programmes for the transition to practice of graduate nurses in New Zealand have been developed and that many of the concerns raised in the present study are being addressed. Of more importance is the preliminary finding that graduates in these programmes are reporting positively on the outcomes.

Nurse Educators

The move of pre-registration nurse education into the polytechs meant that the qualifications of nurse teachers became the focus of much scrutiny. Horsburgh (1996), points out that the polytechs expecting to offer degrees and the New Zealand Qualifications Authority had separately but co-operatively begun to develop criteria relating to the qualifications of teachers in degree programmes. These include the requirement that teaching staff on degree programmes possess qualifications and/or experience at a level higher than the qualification being offered in the degree programme. The author comments:

> Given that the focus of polytechnic degrees must be clinical practice and preparation for clinical practice, it is encouraging to see that experience is an important criterion. I have no anxiety that we have enough teachers who are well prepared, qualified and who have excellent clinical backgrounds to teach in our polytechnic degree programmes (Horsburgh, 1990/91, p. 27).

The author further points out that teaching staff will be expected to undertake research and other scholarly activities, and that such research is likely to be applied rather than esoteric.

Not all writers are so optimistic of the future of nurse educators. One concern expressed by Wilson (1996) for example is that polytechs could begin to cut nursing department staff and hence some nurse teachers could lose their jobs. If this were to happen the author argues, many of these teachers would return to teach students in hospitals, however, this would be at a substantially reduced salary.

Curricular Issues

Sherrard (1995) reports that each polytechnic nursing school has an advisory committee made up of practising nurses who are employed in the local health services. This committee is consulted in all matters relating to the curriculum. The student based courses are termed comprehensive and follow a generalist model, however, Gallagher (1995) indicates that there have been some objections to this approach to nurse education, especially from mental health nurses as they feel that the generalist curriculum does not adequately prepare one for mental health nursing practice. Students learn to adapt and apply basic nursing concepts to all areas of nursing, and the previous distinctions of general nurse, psychiatric nurse etc.... no longer pertain. Clinical practice is co-ordinated with the theoretical component of the course and students receive clinical placements in a diversity of health settings including community health areas (Horsburgh, 1989). The emphasis on community is congruent with international trends in health care provision and policy and is also identified as a curriculum strand by other writers (O'Connor, 1996; Wilson, 1996). Currently it would appear that each polytech school of nursing formulates their own curriculum along broadly similar lines, however, there have been some calls for a national curriculum, this principally due to the small population of the country and the relatively few nurses involved (c N=5000) (Gallagher, 1995).

The Nursing Council continue to approve educational programmes as per the Nurses Act, 1977, however, this pertains to nurse registration only, and is valid for four years.

Sherrard (1995) points out that some nurses are unhappy with this situation as it dilutes the professions ability to determine and monitor its standards of education. Academic approval is the domain of the New Zealand Qualifications Authority (NZQA). In this regard the term approval refers to the written curriculum and supporting documentation for the degree, and according to Sherrard, the process is rigorous and time consuming. This "second stage" approval entails a visit by a panel from the NZQA, whose responsibility it is to recommend the programme for approval or otherwise. The panel comprises eight individuals, including academics from a university who teach in a related discipline, representatives from the nursing profession, an independent chairperson, and a NZQA representative. In order to avoid duplication, the Nursing Council's nurse adviser is both a member of the approval and accreditation panels for nursing and midwifery bachelor degrees. When approval has been granted, the NZQA has a very specific role in monitoring the progress of each degree.

In 1997, the Ministry of Health established a working party to consider issues relating to the mental health component of the under-graduate nursing education programme. The Working party developed mental health criteria for each of 11 generic competencies that had been approved by the Nursing Council in 1996. These mental health criteria were approved by the Nursing Council in November 1997, and the polytechnics are now incorporating the criteria into their programmes.

The 15 nursing programmes and 5 midwifery programmes are audited every three years by the Nursing Council. This is a monitoring process and it is tied into the New Zealand Qualifications Authority (NZQA) monitoring process. The NZQA accredits tertiary institutions, and it is reported that the NZQA and Nursing Council work well together.

Summary

The period between the 1930s and the 1980s was one of continual agitation on the part of nurses for educational reform in nursing in Australia. Nurses were unhappy with their status *vis a vis* other professional workers, and poor pay and conditions were also a source of discontent throughout this period. Like the UK, despite a plethora of reports on the issue, it was not until the early 1980s that the government acceded to significant reforms in this regard. The findings of these official reports represented a severe incrimination of nurse training and graphically emphasised many of the woes that beset nursing at the time. Indeed, in Australia, it took an imminent national nurses strike for which there was considerable public sympathy, before the government agreed to fund the transfer of nursing education to the third level sector. That there was also a chronic high attrition rate in nursing also helped to speed reform.

The initial arrangement was for a three year diploma course. The curriculum was one that offered a comprehensive knowledge base and a reduction in the predominance of the medical model, the award of full student status, an increase in the correlation between theory and practice, and better responsiveness to the ongoing changes in the role of the nurse. It was also prophesised that graduates of the programmes would be competent practitioners who would not alone be equipped with the necessary knowledge, skills and attitudes to provide quality nursing care, but who would also be in a position to shape the healthcare system into the next century. It was also argued that the direction of the nursing programmes in the university setting would assist the development of the discipline of nursing through it's fostering of both research and other academic activity.

The joint ministerial statement of 24th August, 1984, identified the period 1985-1993 as that in which the new diploma programme would be established, however, by 1989, Australian Universities began to phase out sub-bachelor diploma courses. The following year, principally as a result of pressure from within the nursing profession, the government agreed that the initial qualification for registered nurses should be a three year (six semester) bachelors degree, and that this should be achieved by 1992. There were at this time many calls for a four year degree based on the belief that a three year programme was insufficient to allow for adequate theoretical instruction and clinical practice. These calls were denied however, primarily on the grounds of the extra expense that would be incurred by such a development.

Pre-registration nurse education programmes in Australia adopt a generalist model whereby at the end of the programme, graduates are qualified to work in a variety of settings such as general nursing, mental health nursing, children's nursing, elderly care, and community nursing. The goal of this approach is to produce nurses who are capable of functioning in multiple contexts, and the model suggests that discipline maturity occurs after registration. In practice however, there have been a number of difficulties with this model. In particular, studies have shown that the amount of theory and practice hours devoted to mental health nursing varies considerably, and in some cases, no hours are devoted to such studies. This can result in a situation whereby a graduate nurse could find employment in mental health nursing without having had any theoretical instruction or practical experience in the discipline.

Outcome studies of the Australian degree programmes identify a number of issues that are similar to those found in the British outcome studies. For instance, reports suggest that graduates are lacking in clinical competence and organisational skills on first entering professional practice and that they have difficulty relating theory to practice. Indeed, there are reports that for this reason, some graduates find it difficult to seek employment, employers it seems preferring to employ more experienced registered nurses. Notwithstanding this, like their British counterparts, graduate nurses in Australia did not take long to attain a level of clinical competence at least equal to that of the traditionally educated nurses. On the other hand however, outcome studies demonstrate that graduate nurses have a broad theoretical base, are skilled interpersonally, are motivated towards continued professional education, are able to function in a multidisciplinary team, and have an appreciation of the role of research in developing nursing practice.

In an effort to offset graduates apparent initial lack of clinical skills, and in recognition of the relatively short time frame within which to prepare a nurse graduate (3 years), a number of models have been proposed as ones that may assist in graduates transition to practice, including: Graduate Nursing Programmes, Short Orientation Programmes, Preceptorships/Mentorships, and Internships. Despite considerable pressure, the National review on Nurse Education (1994) failed to recommend a four year degree incorporating an internship, principally on the grounds that it would be too costly and also because the committee were of the opinion that the clinical competence of the new graduates could be guaranteed without resorting to an Internship. Furthermore, others were of the view that an Internship was too much like the medical model, and that such an arrangement could merely be regarded as a source of cheap labour for hospitals. Despite these arguments, it would appear that many employers are providing what are described as de-facto internships, the costs of which often are incurred by the graduate nurse. Moreover, it is apparent that many nurses are happy to pay for such programmes as it almost guarantees them a job afterwards.

The move of nurse education to the third level education sector brought about many changes for nurse educators. Indeed, many of these changes are held in common with their British Project 2000 teacher counterparts. For instance, at the time of the transfer, there were insufficient numbers of suitably qualified nurse teachers to develop and teach on the new programmes. Hence, many nurse teachers had to pursue further studies. Unlike the nurse teachers in the UK where it is estimated that only 25% were graduates at the time of the launch of Project 2000, most Australian nurse teachers were graduates, however, the requirement now was that they attain a higher degree at either masters' or doctoral level. The result of this was that pressure was placed on nursing faculties in the universities to facilitate educators to attain such degrees. This created some difficulty for them as there were insufficient higher degree programmes developed at this time. One short term solution was to recruit nursing scholars from North America, New Zealand and the United Kingdom. Australian nurse teachers also experienced an increase in workload and also came under pressure to engage in scholarly activities as part requirement of their university lectureship role. Unlike the UK nurse teachers, between 50-100% of Australian nurse teachers are reported to engage in clinical practice and/or teaching.

Clinical nurse education was the most commonly cited issue of all those raised in submissions to the National review on Nurse Education (1994). Only a modest amount of clinical education was provided for in the first year of the programme, and this gradually increased as the programme progressed. Most schools provide placements in mental health, paediatrics, elderly care and community. Indeed, there is an overall emphasis on a community orientation. However, it is reported that some schools have difficulty in accessing sufficient clinical placements for their students.

Pre-registration nurse education in New Zealand entered the higher education sector long before many of the other countries in the developed world. In 1971, a review of nurse education recommended such a move, and shortly afterwards, this was endorsed by government. There followed a phased transfer, and like it's near neighbour, New Zealand adopts a generalist curriculum model. Clinical placements are provided for in a diversity of settings, however, recently, polytechnics have had to pay for some of these as a result of a shift in government policy. Currently, there is a fear that this extra cost may be shifted onto the already financially stretched student nurse.

Students receive clinical placements in a diversity of settings including mental health and community nursing. Indeed, there is an overall emphasis on community. There are also reports that some disciplines, such as mental health, are not accorded the same weighting in the curriculum, and this has lead to some calls for a return to the old discipline specific approach, whereby there were separate programmes for general, mental health and children's' nursing.

While pre-registration nurse education in New Zealand has not yet moved into the university sector yet, all programmes are located in polytechnics and are at bachelors degree level. Moreover, currently there is considerable debate on this issue, some arguing that pre-registration nurse education should be conducted in universities, while others believe that such a move is premature and therefore potentially harmful to the profession.

CHAPTER 3

CHANGES IN NURSE EDUCATION – CANADA

3.1 A Brief History of Nurse Education

In 1874, nursing education began in Canada with the establishment of the first school of nursing at the General and Marine hospital at St. Catherine's in Ontario. By the turn of the century, twenty more schools had been established in hospitals throughout Canada (Thomas et al., 1992). The first schools were founded very much along the lines of the Nightingale model as was the case in other Commonwealth countries, and nurse training was conducted under an apprenticeship paradigm (Coburn, 1974). Under this model, more emphasis was placed on dedication and on womanly devotion rather than on such educational values as knowledge and critical thinking. Moreover, hospital administrators were soon to realise the advantage of this cheap source of labour and as a result, the number of hospitals offering nurse training grew (Thomas et al., 1992).

In 1919, the first Canadian university based education programme in nursing was established at the University of British Columbia, this principally as a result of the findings of an expert committee established five years earlier. This committee had the specific remit of investigating nursing education and concluded that hospital based training programmes were needlessly laborious, and hence, it was recommended that nurse education be transferred to the educational system (Gibbon and Mathewson, 1947). This first degree programme became the archetype for subsequent nursing degree programmes in Canada and took the form of a "sandwich model." In this model, students enrolled in the university for one year for non-nursing courses and then moved to a hospital-based programme for the nursing component. A fifth year at the university completed the programme. The university had control over the academic portion of the programme and awarded the degree while the hospital controlled the nursing component (French, 1992). King (1970) reports that little co-ordination occurred between these two components of the programme.

In 1932, a survey was undertaken of nursing education in Canada, one of the main recommendations of which was that nurses ought to be given a liberal education as well as a technical education, and that the university based programmes should award participants degrees (French, 1992).

The first truly integrated nursing degree programme was offered in 1942 at the University of Toronto. All nursing courses in this programme were designed to university standard and entrants to the programme had to fulfil normal university entry criteria (Thomas et al., 1992). In these programmes, most of which spanned four academic years, the university had complete control over all of the educational components and as recommended above, the students received both a liberal and a professional education (French, 1992). While the university nursing programmes were popular, integration of nursing education into the higher education system was slow and the vast majority of entrants to the nursing profession continued to enrol in hospital based courses (Hill and Kirkwood, 1991). In the late 1950s, a study commissioned by the Canadian Nurses Association uncovered evidence of varying standards of practice and education and recommended therefore that a process of accreditation of schools of nursing was necessary if standards of education were to be upheld. The report also argued that as long as hospitals held control over schools of nursing, the main focus of student nurse training would remain on service commitment and not on education. Further criticism of the apprenticeship system came in 1964 when the Report of the Royal Commission on Health Services was published. It recommended the expansion of nursing education into universities, the transfer of diploma schools from hospitals to post-secondary educational institutions, and a move from non-integrated nursing degrees (Thomas et al., 1992). It was almost ten years later before the first major response to these recommendations came. In 1973, the provincial government of Ontario announced its intention to move all diploma schools of nursing under the control of the College of Applied Arts and Technology. Similarly, at about the same time in Quebec, hospital schools of nursing closed and nursing programmes were transferred to community colleges. Many other Provinces soon followed suit resulting in a situation whereby pre-registration nurse education was now being offered in a diversity of settings (Thomas et al., 1992), however, French (1992) reports that in the mid 1970s, most diploma nursing programmes were being conducted in community colleges.

Baumgart and Kirkwood (1990) argue that the admission of nursing students to universities was not originally based on developing nursing's scientific knowledge base. Rather it was more often based on a need for public service. This is a view with which Field (1989) concurs, this latter author suggesting that for some time nurse educators remained unconvinced of the need for educational reform in nursing. Indeed the author argues that many nurses were reluctant to give up the traditional three year hospital school of nursing based diploma programmes for the new style of education. Moreover Field argues, when change did come, it was often abrupt, imposed by politicians, and with insufficient planning time to make it a success (Field, 1989). Similarly, Baumgart and Kirkwood (1990) suggest that there was a lot of disagreement as to whether or not nursing should relocate alongside other disciplines in the university setting.

Notwithstanding the fact that university nursing programmes have existed since 1919, the 27 basic Bachelor of Science (Nursing) programmes in 1992, produce only about 17% of newly registered nurses annually (French, 1992). Degree conversion courses have also existed for many years (since early 1920s) and these produce another 1,065 graduates at bachelor's degree level annually (Canadian Association of University Schools of nursing, CAUSN, 1991). According to French in 1992, only 20% of registered nurses are prepared at baccalaureate level or higher. Enrolments in university schools are still low in comparison to those in diploma programmes (Thomas et al., 1992).

3.2 The Need for Change

It can be seen from the foregoing that a gradual momentum for significant educational change in nursing had been building for over half a century. In the early 1980s, Canadian professional nursing associations officially adopted the goal of baccalaureate entry to practice by the year 2000. Since then, nursing educators have explored a variety of means to ensure that this ambition is realised for nursing (Dewis and Grenier, 1993). One of the strongest arguments put forward by nurse educators to move pre-registration nursing education to the university sector was the perceived need for nurses to have a broadly-based education as well as a professional education (French, 1992). This incorporation of liberal education as a component of nursing education was viewed as a means to foster the development of the individual, to prepare the individual for citizenship, to provide the individual with a broad knowledge base, and to develop the individual's critical thinking and judgement skills (Hanson, 1989, 1991). This it was argued could best be achieved through a university education (French, 1992). Similarly, the Alberta Association of Registered Nurses (AARN) in a position paper on graduate education in nursing (1989) argue that more nurses must be prepared at a graduate level in nursing. The Association asserts that this position reflects changes that are taking place within the discipline of nursing, the health care system, and society, and is predicated on a number of beliefs including the following:

- Nursing has a societal mandate to provide safe, competent, ethical nursing care. To meet this mandate, knowledge essential to nursing in the clinical, research, educational, and administrative settings must be developed.

- Graduate education in the discipline of nursing, strengthens the individual's ability to practice from a conceptual framework of nursing.

- Knowledge from other disciplines contributes to the development of nursing knowledge.

AARN concludes that in order to contribute to the development of nursing knowledge which is required to achieve excellence in nursing care, advanced nursing knowledge and skill will be required for nurses in clinical practice, education, administration or research. This they state, requires a university education. Further, it is argued that in order to prepare for current and future changes in the health care delivery system, dramatic increases in the numbers of nurses prepared to graduate level (as well as masters and doctorate levels) in the discipline of nursing is required (AARN, 1989).

The necessity to change in accordance with changing societal needs is also identified by other writers as evidence of an urgency to attain higher education for nurses (Wood, 1996; Dewis and Grenier, 1993; French, 1992 and Baines, 1992). French (1992), points out however that in Canada, living in close proximity to the United States of America (USA) has resulted in many ideas and approaches evolving in nursing in the USA being adopted uncritically by Canadian nurses. However, having easy access to graduate nursing education programmes in the USA has provided Canadian nurses with an opportunity to study at graduate level. French implies that it is now time for Canada to develop its own Canadian culture specific nursing graduate programmes. French further argues that nursing is the only health profession in Canada that does not require a degree in the discipline as the entry criterion to professional practice. Even the newly recognised profession of midwifery (a self-regulating profession that includes nurses with midwifery training as well as non-nurse midwives), requires its members to have an under-graduate degree for entry into the profession. The above position pertains, French points out, despite the fact that professional associations in nursing (except Ontario) have achieved consensus on the issue (French, 1992).

Wood (1996), draws attention to the expectation that in 25 years time, over three quarters of all nurses will work in community settings. This, the author contends, will create many opportunities for nurses especially those who wish to work in education or health promotion. In particular, the author draws attention to the possibility of nurses working as autonomous primary health carers to whom patients have direct access. In order to prepare for these eventualities, Wood argues that nurses need to be well prepared and therefore it behoves nurses to press for a baccalaureate degree as entry to practice (Wood, 1996).

Across Canada there has been a dramatic movement away from two and three year college and hospital based diploma programmes in preference for university based nurse education programmes. This trend according to Dewis and Grenier (1993), very much reflects the efforts to achieve the goal set out at the beginning of this section, that of baccalaureate entry to practice by the year 2000. In order to facilitate the realisation of this goal, several Canadian university schools of nursing have developed links or have integrated with college and/or hospital schools of nursing. There is also evidence that the number of applicants to the traditional schools have been declining while those to the university schools have been on the increase (Dewis and Grenier, 1993).

Calls for baccalaureate entry to the profession have not been unopposed (Field, 1989; French, 1992). Field (1989) suggests that the greatest resistance to educational change may come from nurses themselves and that this may result from the lack of flexibility they experienced in their own educational preparation. The author further alludes to government opposition, this principally on the grounds of the financial implications of such change. In anticipation of such opposition from nurses, the Nurses Association of New Brunswick (NANB) (1994), in order to allay the fears of traditionally prepared nurses who feel that new graduate nurses will jeopardise their jobs and promotion opportunities, introduced what they term a "grandfathering clause." This is a provision that allows these nurses the right to practice throughout their careers without the fear that their qualifications will be deemed obsolete. In December 1994, it was announced by the Minister of Advanced Education that the four year baccalaureate will become the new entry point in New Brunswick (NANB, 1994).

Other opposition to baccalaureate status has centred around the belief by some nurses that nursing is a practice based discipline and as such does not require a university education (Yuill, 1995; Grant, 1995). If this is the case, Grant (1995) argues, then nurses would not require degrees because their work would be under the direction of non-nurses, and hence nurses would not need to develop the research based knowledge that is required to improve practice. As a result the author contends, nurses could be replaced by workers who could do the same duties for lower salaries. Similarly, French (1992) points out that a major factor impeding educational reform in Canada has been the divisions within nursing itself. The author suggests that there are both historical and legal reasons for such divisiveness, however, other parties such as politicians and groups representing hospital administration, have used this situation to stifle progress in educational reform. French (1992) describes how nursing has a potentially strong political power force by virtue of its 300,000 members, however, because of the diversity of groups representing nursing and differing opinions regarding change, this power has been diluted and hence progress has been stifled. The author cites the example of the nursing labour union in Ontario which because it represents in excess of 46,000 nurses, when it opposed baccalaureate entry to nursing, its voice was heard by the policy and decision makers.

3.3 Nursing in Higher Education

The process of moving nursing into higher education in Canada is a complex one chiefly as a result of the fact that so many different provinces and governments are involved. Further, a number of examples of transfer processes are available in the literature (Goldenberg, et al., 1995; Dewis and Grenier, 1993; Baines, 1992). In this section, some of the broader issues relating to the transfer and to the organisation and roles of nursing schools in universities will be discussed. In doing this, some examples of actual transfer arrangements will be given.

In Canada, education is under provincial jurisdiction with federal government supporting higher education through transfer payments. Although there are differences between the provinces in terms of arrangements for nurse education, in most cases a binary system exists (French, 1992). French points out that the standard situation is two distinctive domains with clearly defined mandates, namely, universities and community colleges. Community colleges' mandate tends to vary across the provinces, however, they do not grant degrees. The author cites the example of Ontario where community colleges were set up as terminal education providers in the applied arts and technology sectors. They were not intended to be feeders for the universities. Conversely, in Alberta, collaboration between the two sectors in this regard was encouraged (French, 1992).

In some provinces, a third type of educational institution exists, namely, polytechnic institutes. These institutes offer both undergraduate degree and diploma programmes, and are somewhat akin to the former Colleges of Advanced Education (CAE) in Australia, however, these CAEs are more closely aligned to universities than are Canadian Polytechnical institutes (French, 1992). In Ontario, the role of the community colleges was reviewed in the early 1990s. It was agreed that the binary system of education should remain, however, the taskforce concerned did recommend better collaboration between the universities and the community colleges and greater ease of entry to universities for college graduates (French, 1992).

One example of such a college-university collaboration was given by Baines (1992), an Associate Dean of Nursing at Cariboo College, Kamloops, British Columbia. The example concerns the former hospital based diploma in nursing programme at Kamloops Hospital, British Columbia, which in the 1970s transferred to a local community college (Cariboo College). In the 1980s, the programme was lengthened from the existing two calendar years to three academic years. By the end of that decade, a degree programme for registered nurses had been developed in conjunction with the University of Victoria, and at the time of writing, Baines (1992) reports that Carriboo College is collaborating with four other institutions in developing a generic baccalaureate pre-registration programme in nursing. This programme is integrated with programmes available at the University of Victoria, Camosun College in Victoria, Malaspina College in Nanaimo, and Okanagan College in Kelowna, and allows students a number of options. Firstly, they can exit the programme when they reach diploma level, or secondly, they can continue to complete their Baccalaureate in Nursing (BN). Further, holders of diploma's in nursing from other institutions can enrol and complete their BN in the present programme. Baines (1992) asserts that the development of the programme from hospital based diploma to university based degree can be summarised in three words, namely, vision, will, and readiness.

The final transition to degree status began with a survey of post-basic education needs for practising nurses within the region. The findings of this survey strongly suggested that access to a degree in nursing was a priority of the majority of respondents. Thereafter, the Department of Nursing at Cariboo College approached three universities in the region to discuss the possibility of establishing a degree programme in nursing. The process was suddenly and unexpectedly speeded up when at the same time that the University of Victoria and its school of nursing had agreed to support the initiative, the Ministry of Advanced Education published the results of study on access to university education in the province. The findings of this study suggested that access to degree completion opportunities was needed in places other than Vancouver and Victoria. As a result, the Ministry announced its support for appropriate programmes in this regard and provided funding to Cariboo and the two other colleges to offer degree programmes in five different areas including nursing (in co-operation with the University of Victoria).

A team of programme planners from the college formed a degree completion steering committee, and were released from other duties to work full-time on the degree curriculum and its implementation. The team worked in collaboration with the other colleges and the university. Baines (1992) describes the planning process as "overwhelming" at times with many meetings to attend with individual faculty members, department heads and administrative personnel from all institutions concerned. The author identifies three ingredients which successfully sustained the negotiations, namely: good working relationships, mutual trust and respect, and open communication between the parties involved. It soon became apparent however that the development of a post-registration degree was secondary to the need to develop a pre-registration generic baccalaureate degree.

A number of difficulties arose during the process. Some centred on the fact that both the university and the college had different philosophies. The universities overall aim was seen as the need to advance learning, disseminate knowledge, and to facilitate the intellectual, social, physical and moral development of the student. The colleges philosophy on the other hand was to respond to the educational needs of the community, by offering comprehensive and varied programmes thus expanding students capacity for responsible studentship, vocational competence, and intellectual and social growth. "Respect of these differences and the commitment to maintain university standards helped the two institutions achieve compromises and resolve conflicts" (p. 18). Other problems arose in the admission procedures of both institutions and the need to marry the two, and also in their respective workloads. Because of the universities academic activity requirement of its staff, the number of teaching hours for those teaching the degree programme was less than that for those teaching on the diploma programme. This lead to a perceived elitism in favour of those nurse educators teaching the degree programme, a situation that Baines (1992) points out was unhealthy, particularly as both groups of teachers belonged to the same department. Scholarly activity requirement became another contentious issue. The main focus of the college was on teaching and learning, thus relegating scholarly activity into a secondary position. Conversely, the university sees such activity as an integral part of its faculty. This situation posed a challenge to the college to try and develop and support academic activity within the parameters of its available resources.

The disparity in qualifications of staff between both institutions was seen to further compound the difficulty with perceived elitism. The university requires doctoral level preparation for permanent positions, however, because few of the college's staff held such degrees, the university agreed to allow masters degrees as the minimum qualification in the case of nursing full-time on-going positions. The problem lay in the fact that many of those teaching in the diploma programme were educated to baccalaureate level only and hence were not allowed to teach on the degree programme. This Baines (1992) reports resulted in a marked rift between staff at both institutions. Difficulties also arose in regard to academic freedom. Baines asserts that normally, established academics have the freedom to change courses based on student feedback and their own expertise. This was not possible in the programme described by Baines due to it's collaborative nature, hence, all partners had to agree to any revisions. A further development as a result of the new programme was the appointment of an Associate Dean, a new position that was created by the college, with overall responsibility for the degree programme. Similarly, a position of outreach co-ordinator was also established, the holder being responsible for the co-ordination of the degree programme at the collaborative institutions. What was perhaps the biggest challenge for both institutions was the need to move from a unilateral decision making process to an inter-institutional process. This the author points out was very much facilitated by the good working relationships that both the dean and the programme co-ordinator established.

There were also fiscal implications to the move, and not just in terms of extra resources, salary and workload adjustments, but also in terms of a number of new posts that had to be created such as those of programme director, degree programme admissions officer, clinical placement co-ordinator, and extra support staff. This was managed by first of all assessing existing resources, maximising those available, and adding those that were needed, all the time being mindful of the need to uphold university expectations and standards. Finally Baines (1992) indicates how some students were confused about the roles of the two institutions. They are admitted to Cariboo College, however, they receive their degree from the University of Victoria. Further, the curriculum belongs to the university but is taught by the nurse educators at the college.

A number of other difficulties are reported in the literature concerning the transfer of nursing courses into the university sector. Field (1989) points out that in Alberta, where the goal is a baccalaureate degree as entry to practice by the year 2000, it transpired that many RNs were unable to travel to either of the three university centres as they were married with family commitments, some living in remote rural areas and married to farmers. Clearly for these nurses relocation was unrealistic, and travelling long distances to university on a regular basis was also not possible. Others it was discovered, were unable to live without a salary for a whole year while they studied at the university.

Beaton (1990), identifies four major problems which need to be addressed before university nursing programmes can become properly established. These are:

- an inadequate funding infrastructure,

- insufficient numbers of appropriately prepared nursing faculty,

- lack of consensus on what constitutes graduate education in nursing,

- multiple jurisdictions (e.g.: professional V academic) to which nursing must respond.

The author further poses a number of questions which the profession must address, namely, should the dictates of academia determine the scope and nature of nursing programmes? and should the needs of the practice setting determine the structure and content of graduate curricula? The author contends that there are no easy answers, however, she does urge collaboration, "among graduate faculty, between faculty and students, between academia and the practice setting, among graduate programs across the country and among our nursing organisations." (Beaton, 1990, p. 32).

According to French (1992), the usual pattern in North America is to push for independent faculty status for nursing as quickly as possible. This presents nursing with the challenge to develop further its academic base, while at the same time working collaboratively with other disciplines either across faculties, or as part of the same faculty. The author further asserts that working together to achieve mutual goals as well as discipline specific goals, is often arduous as demonstrated in the example above. It requires that each party respects the autonomy and the stage of development of the other, and that both parties work towards the further development of all. Moreover, it also requires the identification of goals, the aligning of discipline and faculty goals, and the development of an organisational structure that will facilitate the realisation of the goals of each discipline, of faculty, and of the university (French, 1992).

3.4 Curricular Issues

A number of issues concerning undergraduate pre-registration nursing curricula have already been alluded to in this chapter. In this section some of these issues will be further developed.

To become a registered nurse in Canada, the individual may take either a two to three year diploma programme through a hospital or college school of nursing, or a four year university degree programme. (National Review, 1994). Furthermore, all schools are currently working towards a baccalaureate degree as the sole entry criterion for nursing by the year 2000 (AARN, 1989). A number of curriculum models are in operation. However, it would appear that the majority of pre-registration degree programmes adopt a generalist model, one which aims to prepare beginning nurses for a diversity of clinical settings. French (1992) points out that there is much pressure to move towards a model that will prepare "specialists" for the various nursing disciplines separately, however, the basic or four year programmes have resisted that pressure. Some allow students in their final year to select a specialist area to concentrate on (French, 1992), and a number of programmes offer a dual exit option. After three years the student can exit the programme with a diploma, or after a fourth year, can exit with a baccalaureate degree (Goldenberg et al., (1995).

Smadu (1995) examines the role of competencies in nurse education and in doing so identifies a number of issues that need to be taken into consideration by curriculum planners in preparing nurses for future nursing practice. These include the implications of health care reform, changes in nursing education, the advent of the information age, advancements in technology particularly in medicine, the concept of the world as a global village, an increased emphasis on primary health care, and changing patterns of illness and health.

Smadu (1995) argues that health care reforms are having a significant effect on the role of the nurse and the scope of practice. In Canada's changing health environment, the expectations of the registered nurse are increasing, including both an expansion of current competencies and the learning of new competencies. Ross (1995) points out that Canadian nurses are now being recognised as the logical care-givers to provide primary health care, and that expanded roles for nurses are finally being legitimised in this regard. Similarly, Wood (1996) suggests that with the move towards community health-based care, there will be more and more opportunities for nurses to set up nurse-run community health centres. The author identifies two major issues that need to be addressed before such a radical but logical change in nursing work can come to fruition. Firstly, there is a need for nurses to be appropriately educated for such future challenges, and secondly, the issue of access to nursing services must be addressed. Simard (1992) describes the impact of health care reform in Saskatechewan and in particular the impact the developing wellness model of care will have on nursing:

> Nurses will increasingly be the primary health team members in many communities, working in partnership with medical and other professionals and assuming other expanded roles where required. A greater primary health care role for public health nurses, and mental health, rehabilitation and other community health workers will be encouraged (Simard, 1992, p. 20).

Smadu (1995) identifies two issues relating to the implications of change in nursing curricula. One, the move to baccalaureate as entry to practice has already been discussed above. The other is the effects of the "curriculum revolution." Smadu (1992) reported that a common thread in the literature on the curriculum revolution is that nursing education programmes need to be changed in terms of content, process, and outcomes, this in order to ensure that future nursing graduates are adequately prepared to practice as registered nurses within a reformed health care system in a continually changing world. The author identifies what she sees as the key features of the curriculum revolution, namely, caring as the essence of nursing practice; the empowerment of clients, students and faculty; an emphasis on critical thinking and clinical judgement; an acknowledgement of a variety of ways of knowing; critical social theory; and phenomenology. Other authors have similarly identified a number of key features of the curriculum revolution. For example, Wood (1996) identifies such factors as problem solving, critical analytical thinking, a community focus, and independent learning, while Field (1989) suggests that computer skills will be essential in the future. Related to this, the author asserts that computer assisted learning will have a part to play in nursing education, however, points out that while computers will provide a most flexible and accepted means of continued study in the future, nursing is grounded in caring, something that cannot be taught by a machine. The author argues therefore that "we must balance the advantages of the mechanised learning with the role model of the caring teacher-learner encounter" (p. 293). Field also identifies lifelong learning, and the skills of learning how to learn as other important curricular issues that need to be considered. Moreover, the author contends that above all the student needs to be cared for throughout the curriculum, as "students who are not cared for will be unable to give care to others" (p. 294). Indeed Dolan (1993) points out that nursing curricula in Canada have gradually moved away from an emphasis on psychomotor (doing) skills in favour of cognitive (knowing) skills since the 1960s.

With regard to collaboration in curriculum development, Field (1989) suggests that clinical nurse experts must work with faculty in developing any blueprint for the future. Educational institutions must include senior hospital and community nursing staff on curriculum planning committees and openly examine the needs and the way in which education can be offered to produce a viable graduate. Clinical nursing practice that is likely to motivate staff towards continued learning and which will enhance skills must also be investigated as part of the curriculum process. This is important the author argues if efforts to keep expert nurses at the patents bedside are to succeed (Field, 1989).

3.5   Issues in Funding

Funding for nursing in Canada has traditionally been a function of joint federal/state arrangements (Shorten and McMurray, 1992). In addition to these central funds, students also pay tuition fees (Dewis and Grenier, 1993).

Beaton (1990) reports how unlike disciplines such as medicine and engineering, funding infrastructure for nursing education is underdeveloped in the university sector. This is further compounded by government cuts in funding, and the author asserts, has had grave implications for the developing graduate programmes in nursing. In times of funding cuts, governments and universities are understandably reluctant to embark on new programmes of study. Nursing, as one of the most recent disciplines to enter the university sector, has been hindered in its development as a result. Moreover, faculties and schools of nursing in some cases have been known to redirect internal funding to these fledgling nursing degree programmes (Beaton, 1990).

Fortunately for some faculties/schools of nursing, initial set-up funding has been provided by state government in order to assist in the establishment of the collaborative arrangements with the universities (Goldenberg et al., 1995; Baines, 1992). However, Beaton (1990) warns that there is no guarantee that this special funding will continue, or that it will remain protected from university cut backs. Beaton further points out that because inadequate funding of graduate education has gone on for so long, a serious shortage of faculty staff with the necessary academic qualifications to teach in these graduate nursing programmes has occurred.

While it would appear that some students qualify for student scholarships or sponsorships, or take out a student loan, Wall (1991) points out that many have to resort to family resources to finance their nursing education. This can become particularly burdensome when one considers such extra costs as uniforms, costs of tuition, and books, as well as a number of hidden costs such as photocopying, parking or bus fare, exam fees and registration fees, the author argues. Funding ones nursing education becomes more complex if one is a mature student and has family commitments as is often the case (Beaton, 1990). Moreover, Field (1989) asserts that in many cases undergraduate bursaries were inadequate. French (1992) points out that for RNs pursuing a degree in nursing, it could take the student 45 years to make up salary lost through leaving the workforce to study full-time for two years, even if the nurse worked between academic sessions and during holidays.

3.6   Implications for Nurse Educators

Perhaps the single most important factor for nurse educators in Canada when colleges of nursing developed collaborative links with universities was that of the need to upgrade qualifications. Indeed, a number of reports have suggested that many nurse educators from the community colleges were lacking in the academic qualifications that were required to work in the university sector (Baines, 1992, French, 1992; Beaton, 1990). It has already been described earlier in this chapter how educators who did not have doctoral degrees were often "relegated" to a role primarily concerned with teaching and learning activities, and were less likely to be privy to engage in more scholarly activities (Baines, 1992).

Another consequence of this shortage of adequately prepared academic staff according to Beaton, (1990) is that faculty must often perform under excessive administration and supervisory workloads. This extra workload consequently interrupts their scholarly activities and perhaps of greater concern, prohibits them from providing intellectual leadership to the profession.

In 1989, the AARN highlighted the need for nurse educators to upgrade to graduate status and to attain masters and doctoral degrees, this in anticipation of the changes that were to come about in the 1990s. Moreover, the Nursing Association of New Brunswick (NANB) (1994) at the time that funding was announced for a new baccalaureate undergraduate degree, stated that a critical factor in the success of this transition would be the upgrading of qualifications for nurse educators. Another factor of note in this regard is that universities take staff qualification profiles into consideration when approving new academic programmes. While there is evidence that a concerted effort was being made to increase the amount of nurse educators who were qualified to doctoral level (French, 1992), access to PhD education in nursing was not easy. Estimates are that in 1989, the majority of nurses with doctorates, held them in non-nursing disciplines (CAUSN, 1991). Beaton (1990) agrees that opportunities for nurses to obtain doctoral degrees in nursing in Canada are rare. This has been complicated by the fact that masters degree programmes and the development of doctoral education has been profoundly influenced by the limited supply of nurses with graduate preparation. The author points out that only 19% of those 193 nurses who earned doctorates in Canada, have a doctorate in the discipline of nursing.

That nursing entered academe late also presented problems for nurse educators during the transfer to the university setting. In many ways this was unavoidable as there were relatively few university nursing departments (schools/faculties), also, nursing is young in comparison to the broader scientific community, and as indicted above, most nurse teachers in the community colleges were educated to baccalaureate level only. Furthermore, a necessary delay for nurses in advancing their academic qualifications is the fact that most nurse academics must spend many of their early professional years gaining clinical experience. (Becker, 1995). One obvious consequence of all of this is that nurse educators were lacking in academic qualifications when the move to the universities came about, but also, such scholarly pursuits as research activity and academic publications remained underdeveloped (Becker, 1995; French, 1992).

An example of the effects of a hospital diploma school-university school collaboration on nurse educators is given by Dewis and Grenier, (1993). The authors describe the model of collaboration between a university school (University of British Columbia-UBC), and a hospital based school (Vancouver General Hospital-VGH) in developing a baccalaureate under-graduate programme. In this collaboration, each partner remained the employer of its own teaching staff, and all nurse educators employed by VGH were given joint appointments as university clinical associates. At the time of the collaboration, 40% of the VGH educators held a masters degree or were in the process of completing one, while the remainder held baccalaureate degrees. At the end of the first programme cycle, the authors point out that at least a masters degree is now required for newly employed faculty, and all new appointments to the VGH faculty are made in consultation with the director of the university school of nursing. Prior to the transition to the baccalaureate programme, all VGH faculty were released from their responsibilities in the diploma programme, and were given a three month orientation to the baccalaureate programme and its curriculum. The authors further report that within two years of the commencement date, all VGH faculty had been "phased into" the new programme, and all are teaching throughout the four years of the programme (Dewis and Grenier, 1993). Dewis and Grenier, (1993) further identify a number of personal and professional concerns expressed by both VGH and UBC faculty at the time of the transition. The most commonly expressed personal concerns were to do with fears of threatened job security, inadequate academic qualifications, inadequate skills to perform in a different teaching role, increased role demands and, disruption of established working relationships. UBC faculty concerns focused on increased workloads as a result of larger enrolments, and also the fear of being outnumbered in decision making. University sessional staff were particularly concerned about their jobs, some fearing that the VGH staff would replace them. While UBC staff supported the principles and goals of the collaboration, they did express concerns that the quality of the educational experience of the student might be compromised. In particular, the UBC staff expressed concern at the pedagogical orientation of the diploma school staff and also questioned their readiness to teach on an academic programme that "aimed to foster analytical and critical thinking, independent and self-reliant learning, theory based nursing, creativity, scholarship, reflection, inquiry, and moral and ethical awareness" (Dewis & Grenier, 1993, p. 1018). The VGH faculty on the other hand, feared the loss of valuable acute care clinical learning experiences. Concerns were also expressed on both sides at the anticipated loss of their respective schools' identities.

Another issue of contention was the fact that the hospital faculty had to travel more often than did the university faculty, this by virtue of the fact that the majority of courses were based on the university campus. This meant that hospital faculty had to plan extra time in their schedule to allow for travel and also, it meant extra expense for the hospital. The university on the other hand had difficulty providing office space for the hospital faculty. Further, while the VGH staff were included in decision making, some problems arose in regard to course involvement and year co-ordination and administration. Dewis and Grenier (1993) report that the issue of identity and equality of partnership also required ongoing commitment on both sides.

It would also appear that each group had different work priorities. University faculty workloads not alone concerned teaching on the undergraduate programme, but also included such scholarly activity as ongoing research and publishing. VGH faculty on the other hand seemed to value more their teaching and learning mission. Scholarly activities were seen as being of less importance. Moreover, the authors reported that hospital faculty were initially concerned that they would be expected to undertake the greater part of the teaching in order to allow university faculty to pursue scholarly activities. This however was not the case.

University teaching staff tend to be more autonomous and independent in their work, and very much value this. This type of work culture the authors contend, does not fit well with collaborative endeavours of this nature, nor to the possibility of increased structural and external direction. On the contrary, VGH staff were accustomed to such a work model. Hence, VGH staff had some difficulty with the amount of autonomy and responsibility that was expected of them after the transfer.

The issue of disparity in salaries between the two groups was also addressed by the authors. The VGH faculty were union members and as such their conditions of employment were determined according to a contract agreed upon between their employer and their union. The university faculty were non-unionised, however, salary differences it would appear did not cause a problem in the working relationships of the two groups. Furthermore in this regard, negotiations with the VGH faculty unions regarding the need to have more flexibility in the work week also became necessary.

Dewis and Grenier (1993) identify three main strategies which they believe sustained the collaborative effort. Great efforts were made to maintain open communication and to keep all staff informed. Open forums were established in the first year, both in the hospital and the university, and later, involving both groups together. Joint team meetings also contributed significantly to providing opportunities for staff to get to know each other and to develop respect for and trust in each others talents and strengths. The promotion of faculty development was seen as requiring urgent attention. Orientation programmes were established to facilitate staff from both sites to get to know the curriculum and to adjust to their new roles and responsibilities. VGH staff were given the opportunity to advance their curriculum development skills by taking on projects such as the development of elective courses, or the participation in curriculum related research projects. A research committee was established in the hospital school during the first year of the programme, this to enable teachers to utilise more research in teaching. The authors assert that this development has been successful in increasing the knowledge and awareness of faculty about research. Furthermore, several of the hospital faculty were reported to be involved in university school research projects. The final strategy that was identified by Dewis and Grenier (1993) is that of maintaining a positive climate. The authors noted that at the outset, some staff on both sides were using inappropriate coping mechanisms to deal with the stress of the change process. These included stereotyping and scapegoating. The result of these behaviours was an increase in tensions between the two groups. In order to prevent such behaviours damaging the process, great efforts were made to establish and develop trust through the communication of potentials and the discussion of feelings at the open forums.

While the authors accept that the organisation and implementation of such joint ventures will be different elsewhere, the model of collaboration presented has much to offer to any similar such project. Dewis and Grenier (1993) conclude that while the decision to work together involved a high degree of risk, taking advantage of the opportunity and managing it well has resulted in professional gains for both parties, and ultimately has benefited consumers of nursing and health care.

3.7   Outcomes of Nurse Education

Proposed Outcomes of Graduate Nurse Education

A number of goals have been set out by various authors for the Canadian university diploma and baccalaureate programmes. Indeed some of these goals and their philosophical underpinnings have already been mentioned in this chapter. The AARN (1989) in its position paper on graduate nurse education suggest that significant numbers of nurses must be prepared to graduate level and that these nurses should be able to provide nursing care at an advanced level, conduct nursing research to provide knowledge for nursing practice, provide basic and continuing nursing education, and administer nursing practice in clinical settings. Similarly, Smadu (1995) identifies a number of competencies required of the modern day nurse. These the author argues are necessarily different from the competencies required in the past, as today's nurse must occupy a diversity of roles such as advocate, teacher, counsellor, and co-ordinator of patient care, as well as roles concerning nursing's work with developing communities. The competencies that Smadu identifies include caring, knowing the patient, critical thinking, clinical judgement, patient teaching and interdisciplinary collaboration. Smadu cites Tanner in this regard, the latter author suggesting that the outcomes of contemporary nursing education programmes should be "caring, critically thinking nurses who can safely practice in both today's world of high-tech disease care and tomorrow's world of true health care." (Tanner, 1990, p. 298).

Advantages of the actual experience of engaging in collaborative initiatives between hospital based schools of nursing and university schools of nursing have also been outlined in the literature. Dewis and Grenier (1993) in the paper discussed in the previous section, identified a number of such advantages. The successful, and sometimes difficult, process that these authors described resulted in an increase in the overall number of graduate enrolments in the baccalaureate programme, thus increasing the numbers of nurses holding baccalaureate degrees in the province. Furthermore, the university school of nursing has through the collaboration initiative, gained valuable access to a wide variety of excellent clinical resources. Not alone are these clinical resources available for the curriculum, but also for summertime work-study projects and independent guided studies. Moreover, the authors point out that the university has also gained access to the diploma school faculty's clinical and teaching expertise. The gains to the development of nursing research are also catalogued. The human, financial and physical resources of both schools are available to all, and the opportunities for creative and innovative endeavours through the reciprocal access to the expertise within each faculty has enhanced nursing research efforts. In addition the authors point out, the collaboration will continue to assist the hospital to develop as a centre of excellence, which in turn it is argued, will enable it to attract and retain highly qualified nurses.

Exit Characteristics and Outcomes after Graduation

While there is a dearth of research literature on the outcomes of pre-registration nurse education programmes in Canada, there is some anecdotal evidence that suggests that beginning nurses are not always ready for their staff nurse role (Yuill, 1995; Melchior-Mac Dougall, 1992) For example, Melchior-MacDougall (1992) suggest that a common complaint of nurse employers is that graduates do not have the clinical skills required to practice competently in acute care settings. The authors go on to describe an educational programme (in addition to the pre-registration programme, that is in effect an internship), the express aim of which is to improve the clinical and other practice skills of the beginning nurse.

Dyck, et al., (1991) examined the personal preference characteristics of students entering a baccalaureate nursing programme in Western Canada in order to assist the faculty in planning a relevant curriculum. The authors assert that, in order to achieve nursing education goals, student characteristics should be taken into consideration when planning and implementing a curriculum. If for example the nursing programme aims to produce nurses who are independent, visionary leaders, then it is important to determine if students entering the programme have an interest in being change agents and possess the characteristics of autonomy and dominance. If they do not possess these characteristics, then the authors argue, a system of challenges and rewards for such behaviours must be incorporated into the curriculum as a integral part of the professionalisation process. Dyck et al., (1991) using an non-experimental pre-test, post-test design, administered the Edwards Personal Preference Schedule (EPPS), a classic personality test designed primarily as a research instrument, which provides measures of 15 relatively independent normal personality variables. This tool was chosen as it has well established reliability and validity, and is easy to administer. Seventy two out of a class of 80 first year nursing students entered the study, representing a 90% participation rate. Of these however, only 38 students completed both the pre-and post test questionnaire accounting for an 86% response rate of the 44 eligible students. Students recorded their responses to the EPPS during their second week in the programme and again during the final month of their fourth year.

Table 3.1 shows the mean scores on the EPPS of the first year students compared with the college norm. It can be seen from the table that nursing students scored lower than the norm on such attributes as achievement, deference, autonomy, dominance and change, while higher scores were recorded for order, affiliation, succorance, nurturing and endurance. Indeed, these attributes are consistent with the stereotypical image of the nurse the researchers argue.

TABLE 3.1.   Mean scores on EPPS of 1st year nursing students as compared with the college norm

Variable	Nursing student Mean*	College Norm Mean**	Nursing student S.D.	College Norm S.D.	tvalue
Achievement	12.72	13.08	4.27	4.19	0.69
Deference	11.88	12.40	3.11	3.72	1.33
Order	11.04	10.24	3.76	4.37	1.70
Exhibition	14.07	14.28	3.36	3.65	0.50
Autonomy	11.43	12.29	4.14	4.34	1.67
Affiliation	18.08	17.40	4.50	4.07	1.24
Intraception	16.96	17.32	4.54	4.70	0.64
Succorance	14.38	12.53	4.55	4.42	3.30
Dominance	11.17	14.18	4.54	4.60	5.38
Abasement	15.99	15.11	4.62	4.94	1.54
Nurturing	19.67	16.42	4.60	4.41	5.75
Change	16.07	17.20	4.23	4.87	2.13
Endurance	14.39	12.63	4.15	5.19	3.36
Heterosexuality	11.92	14.34	4.86	5.39	3.99
Aggression	10.10	10.59	3.32	4.61	1.15

xf**n=72
**n=749.

Source: **Dych et al, 1991.**

The findings reported by Dych et al (1991) suggest that some changes may have occurred in the student population over the course of the study, particularly in relation to the characteristics of achievement and autonomy. While respondents were still scoring lower than the college norm on these characteristic, the differences were not found to be statistically significant. Dych and colleagues also noted a continued low scoring for dominance at the end of year four, the researchers noting that this finding was in tandem with those of other studies of this nature. This was also true for the characteristic of nurturance, for which it was found there was a high need. It was also evident from the data that there was a high need in this cohort for succorance, a trait that received inconsistent scoring among nursing students in other studies. The finding of a lower need for affiliation at the end of year four may be better understood if one considers the possibility that at the time of the first EPPS scoring (2 weeks into the programme), most of the students were likely to have been ill at ease and looking for new friendships in order to survive. By the end of the fourth year however, it is likely that students were more confident and had developed many friendships and relationships.

On the whole Dych et al (1991) report that no major shifts in these personality characteristics occurred for students over the course of the four years. The researchers note that this seems to suggest that the students had assimilated into the college norm by the time of graduation. Notwithstanding this, Dych et al (1991) contend that even though there were no significant differences found, their findings still have implications for curriculum planning. For example, the researchers point out that the students need for nurturance is perhaps a desirable characteristic as in the words of Newton (1981, p. 353): "Only the nurse makes the system morally tolerable," the author here referring to the ever increasing technical and bureaucratic health care system. However, a challenge for curriculum planners according to Dych et al (1991), is to blend this traditionally feminine nurturing role with more masculine values such as autonomy, scholarly research, and scientific problem solving. Moreover, the profession seeks to convey an image and a reality of autonomy and leadership. Hence, the curriculum must be designed to foster such traits and prepare nurses to be innovative in their approach to nursing situations. To achieve this with nurses who have a low need for dominance and change necessitates specifically designed learning activities. The researchers identify a number of teaching strategies that contribute to these goals including, independent study, case studies, student presentations, and debates. Similarly, with regard to students low need for change, Dych and colleagues suggest that teachers must model and teach change processes and identify the need for change in the profession. The authors conclude that through recognition of natural tendencies and cultural stereotypes, it is possible to promote the development of personal characteristics in students that are consistent with the future needs of the nursing profession and the needs of clients.

While it is a moot point, it would appear that the above characteristics should be taken into consideration by those selecting candidates for nurse training, and this is an issue not really addressed by Dych et al (1991) Much effort and expense has been vested in higher education for nurses, especially at baccalaureate level. If it transpires, as appears to be the case here, that little change occurs in these stereotypical nursing traits, perhaps the much hoped for critical thinking, skilled decision making, autonomous, assertive nurse will not emerge from such programmes. Further research is required as a matter of some urgency, to investigate this issue of entry and exit characteristics of nursing students.

Hiscott in 1995 analysed data from the National Graduates Surveys (Statistics Canada), by examining four distinctive cohorts of nursing programme graduates (degree and diploma), between 1978 and 1992. A number of notable trends and patterns were observed from the data. With respect to employment outcomes, the overwhelming majority of nursing graduates (>90%) were employed in clinical nursing two years after graduation. However, it was noted that there was an increase in part-time and temporary employment among nursing graduates. Furthermore, the fact that "unavailability of full-time jobs" was the reason cited for part-time employment suggests that this situation was involuntary and not as a result of personal choice. Hiscott points out also, that this trend in underemployment is not peculiar to nursing graduates.

It also emerged from the nurse data that there was a correlation between completed post-secondary qualifications and success in gaining early career employment, this was much more the case for graduate baccalaureate nurses than for non-degree holding nurses.

Moreover, most nursing graduates were subsequently employed in jobs for which their educational programme was designed, and in positions that utilised their specialist skills. It was also noted from this data that the vast majority of recent graduate suggested that they would choose the same programme of study again, and at the time of the latest survey (1992), approximately four out of five nursing graduates indicated that they would choose the same education programme again.

Summary

Like its other Commonwealth counterparts, historically nurse education in Canada was conducted under the apprenticeship model. In 1919 however, the first Canadian university based education programme in nursing was established. This was as a result of the findings of an expert committee on nursing education which concluded that hospital based training programmes were needlessly laborious, and hence the committee recommended that nurse education be transferred to the general education system. However, while these early degree programmes proved to be popular, integration of nurse education into the higher education sector was slow. The first major move of nurse education did not occur until almost 50 years later when in the early 1970s, most of the hospital based diploma programmes moved into community colleges. Finally in the early 1980s, Canadian professional nursing associations officially adopted the goal of baccalaureate entry to practice by the year 2000.

The main rationale behind this goal was the belief that nurses needed to have a broadly-based as well as a professional education. Moreover, it was felt that the liberal education that would be offered in a baccalaureate degree, would help to foster the development of the individual, and his/her critical thinking and judgement skills. Such a goal was also deemed necessary to prepare the nurse for current and future changes in the health care delivery system. Other's welcomed the move towards degree status as they felt that it would at last redress the unfair situation whereby nurses were the only health professionals who were not educated to degree level. This goal towards degree status was not without opposition. Indeed chief among the detractors were nurses themselves. Some felt that nursing would become too theoretical and that bedside skills would be lost. There was also some government opposition, this principally on the grounds of the financial implications of such a change.

While most schools of nursing in Canada are now moving towards the four year baccalaureate degree, there are still some community colleges offering three year diploma programmes. Indeed, some of the university courses allow students to exit from the programme after three years with a diploma, or else they can remain on for the fourth year and exit with a degree.

A number of curriculum models are in operation, however, it would appear that the majority of pre-registration degree programmes adopt a generalist model, one which aims to prepare beginning nurses for a diversity of clinical settings. There is some evidence of a move towards a return to the traditional approach however. This approach, analogous to the current situation here in Ireland, prepared nurses for distinct disciplines within nursing such as general nursing, sick children's nursing, and so on. So far it would appear that such a move has been resisted.

Nurse educators in Canada were affected by the move to higher education in similar ways to nurse educators elsewhere. Many nurse educators from the community colleges were lacking in the academic qualifications that were required to work in the university

113

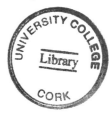

sector. This was complicated by the fact that there were a paucity of doctoral degree programmes in nursing available to them. Traditionally, it would appear that Canadian nurse academics studied for higher degrees in the United States. There is evidence however, that a concerted effort is currently being made to increase the number of nurse educators who are qualified to doctoral level. Other issues that concerned nurse educators involved the fear that some might lose their job security, that they had inadequate skills to perform in a different teaching role, and that their established working relationships would be disrupted. An increase in workload was reported by other nurse teachers.

It would now appear that this new approach to pre-registration nurse education has been accorded much governmental and professional approval, and there is also an acceptance that the generalist graduate nurse of the future is perhaps the most logical person to deliver primary health care.

CHAPTER 4

NURSE EDUCATION – FRANCE

4.1 General Overview of Nurse Education in France

Pre-registration nurse education in France is of three years duration, at the end of which successful students are conferred with a State Nurse's Diploma (DEI). The overall supervision of nurse education in through the Ministry of Health, and is governed by a number of pieces of legislation that are specific to nursing. There is no nursing board as such, however as will be seen below, each training institution has a Board of Studies some of the functions of which are similar to those of national nursing boards in other countries.

Nurse education is conducted in Hospital nurse training schools of which there were 349 in 1996, however, there are also a few universities and lycees involved in nurse education. In general, nursing students are considered to be of similar status as university students (level III). Entrants to nurse training must be 17 years or more and must have completed 12 years of general education. Most hospital schools admit students on the basis of a general knowledge test, psychological tests, and an interview.

There also exists a system of monitoring the quality of educational programmes and this function is exercised through the Health Ministry. This is operationalised through regional and departmental directorates for health and social affairs, and by among others, the presidency of the Technical Council and by other means of monitoring, which takes place at least twice a year.

The course of study spans 4,760 hours over the three years, 2,485 of which are devoted to theoretical instruction. During their studies, students receive a small amount of funding from the training institutions which approximates to about 1,300FF in years two and three. It is unclear to this writer whether or not funding is granted in year one.

4.2 Board of Studies

Each school of nursing is required to establish a Board of Studies or Technical Advisory Council which is to be consulted on all matters relating to the training of students. The Director of the school must submit information pertaining to the curriculum to this Board of Studies, such as teaching arrangements, the aims of the course, the general organisation of studies, information relating to students' supervised work, practicals and clinical placements and the teaching materials in use. Other duties of the Director of the school in this regard are to submit to the Board details of the schools budget, numbers and specialisation of teaching staff, details on student fees for entry tests where applicable, and also students' examination results at the end of the year.

The Bord of Studies of all training schools is established by order of the Prefet, the State's representative at Department of Health level. the Board is chaired by the State's representative or his deputy, and apart from the Director and Technical Director of the School, it includes representatives of the hospitals management body, teachers, and students. Membership of the Board of Studies is outlined in Table 4.1 All of the Boards members have the right to vote on issues that arise. Student representatives are elected for one year while all other members are elected or nominated for a period equal to the duration of the educational programme. Further, the chairperson has the right to request the attendance of any other person at the Board from whom advice is sought.

The Board of Studies is required to hold at least two meetings per year and these are convened by the Director of the school in consultation with the chairperson. A quorum of two thirds is required before a meeting of the Board can be declared valid, if such a quorum is not present the meeting must be postponed and a new meeting must be convened within one week. A this meeting, the Board is considered valid to make decisions no matter how many members are present.

4.3 Nurse Training Institutions

Nurse training institutions are run by a Director who is responsible for syllabus design, organisation of the initial, preparatory and in-service training offered in the institution. He/she also organises theoretical and practical education, checks students' progress, is responsible for the assignment and management of teaching staff, and promotes and participates in research into nursing by teachers of the training institution. The Director is also responsible for the general operation of the institution, including administrative and financial management. He/she is not permitted any other remunerated employment. Directors must fulfil the following requirements:

- Be age thirty or more.

- Hold one of the qualifications mentioned in Article L.474-1 or L.477 of the public health code (? nursing qualification/registration).

- Hold one of the following qualifications:

    — charge nurse certificate,

    — certificate of competence as ward nurse,

    — certificate of competence as supervisory nurse,

    — certificate of competence as public health charge nurse,

    — certificate of supervisor of vocational training for psychiatric nursing staff.

- Have carried out teaching duties in a nurse training institution or in a school for supervisory staff for at least three full years after obtaining whichever nursing qualification is appropriate.

The objectives of the nurse training institution include the initial training of nurses and nursing assistants, preparatory training for entrants, in-service education including re-training, and documentation on and research into nursing.

116

TABLE 4.1. Members of the board of studies

Ex officio members:
- — The State's representative at Department level or deputy Chairperson.
- — The Director of the School of Nursing.

Representatives of management and other suitable individuals:
- — The chair of the Board of Directors of the management organisation.
- — The Director of the management organisation.
- — The Head of Nursing Services in the institution which runs the programme.
- — A doctor or a pharmacist who is resident or involved in management, as proposed by the Board of Directors of the management organisation.
- — nurse working in the community sector (non-hospital) designated by the State's representative in the Department.

Student Representatives:
- — Six student nurses elected by the student body (2 from each year).

Representatives of the Trainers:
- — Three senior ward nurses taking part in the training of students in the training establishment concerned, as elected by their colleagues.
- — Two senior nurses with managerial responsibilities in the nursing service in a health establishment, the first in a public health establishment, the second in a private health establishment, as elected by their colleagues.
- — One doctor elected by colleagues.

Other Members:
- — The regional technical adviser for nursing or the teaching adviser in those regions where there is one.
- — A university lecturer, elected by colleagues, in those cases where the training institution has an agreement with a university.

Source: **Ministere des affaires Sociales de la Sante et de la Ville, 1992.**

4.4   Theoretical and Clinical Education

The senior nurses in training institutions (clinical and management nurses), contribute to the theoretical and clinical teaching under the management of the Director, and are also involved in the clinical assessment of students. They are responsible for keeping track of students academic progress and are expected to participate in nursing research. While the Ministry suggests that the numbers of such personnel shall be sufficient to ensure a satisfactory teacher:student ratio, it is unclear what the ideal or normal ratio is. Ward nurses taking part in training students in a nurse training institution must hold a diploma as State Nurse or State Psychiatric Nurse.

They must also hold one of the following qualifications:

- — charge nurse certificate,

- — certificate of competence as ward nurse,

- — certificate of competence as supervisory nurse,

- — certificate of competence as public health charge nurse,

- — psychiatric charge nurse certificate

- — certificate of supervisor of vocational training for psychiatric nursing staff.

The theoretical classes given to students may be provided by ward nurses participating in training institutions, by nurse managers, by doctors, by pharmacists, and by any other person suitably qualified in the subject concerned. It would appear that there is no grade akin to nurse tutor/nurse teacher per se. Rather much of the teaching is carried out by the above clinical nursing, medical and paramedical staff. Theoretical instruction modules are outlined in Tables 4.2 and 4.3.

TABLE 4.2.   Obligatory theoretical modules (2,080 Hours, 35 Hours per week)

Subject	Modules	Hours
Human Sciences	2	160
Anatomy, Physiology and Pharmacology	1	100
Ethics and Law	1	80
Public Health	1	80
Nursing	4	360
Hygiene	1	60
Nursing care of Patient with infectious diseases and of patient with HIV	1	80
Nursing care of Patient with Cardio-vascular disease	1	60
Nursing care of Patient with Respiratory disease	1	60
Nursing care of Patient with trauma and Orthopaedic disorders	1	60
Nursing care of adolescents, adults and the elderly with psychiatric disorder	4	360
Children's nursing and Child Psychiatry	1	80
Nursing care of Patient with Digestive disorder	1	60
Nursing care of Patient with Endocrine Disorder	1	40
Nursing care of Patient with Renal/Urological Disorder	1	60
Nursing care of Patient with Neurological Disorder	1	60
Nursing care of Patient with Haemopathies and cancer	1	80
Nursing care of Older Patient	1	80
Nursing care of Patient with Blood Transfusion	1	80
Nursing care of Patient with Obstetric/Gynaecological Needs/Disorder	1	40
Nursing care of Patient with Ear/Nose & Throat Disorders, with facio-maxillary surgery, with a Stoma, with Ophthalmic Disorder or with Dermatological Disorder	1	40
Total	28	2,080

Source: **Ministere des affaires Sociales de la Sante et de la Ville, 1992.**

TABLE 4.3.   Optional Theoretical Modules *(Student must choose two modules)*

Subject	Modules	Hours
Nursing care of patient with Cardio-vascular disorder	1	80
Nursing care of patient with Respiratory Disorder	1	80
Nursing care of the trauma/orthopaedic patient	1	80
Nursing care of patient with digestive disorder	1	80
Children's nursing	1	80
Nursing care of adolescent, adult and older person with mental illness I	1	80
Nursing care of adolescent, adult and older person with mental illness II	1	80
Community and Primary Health	1	80
Total	2	160

Source: **Ministere des affaires Sociales de la Sante et de la Ville, 1992.**

The Director of the training institution selects potential clinical placement areas from within public and private health establishments, as well as non-hospital health establishments. He/she must then submit a list of these placement areas to the Inspector of Health for the Department in which the institution is situated. This official, who is a doctor, may exclude from this list any establishments which are deemed to be unsuitable for the purposes of student nurse clinical training. Clinical placements for the diploma course are set out in Table 4.4.

TABLE 4.4. Clinical placements *(2,275 Hours, 35 Hours per week)*

Disciplines	Weeks	Hours
1st Year		
Medicine	4	140
Mental Health & Psychiatry	4	140
Geriatrics/Psycho-Geriatrics	3	105
Public Health	3	105
Surgery	4	140
Total 1st Year	**18**	**630**
2nd Year		
Medicine	4	140
Surgery	4	140
Psychiatry/Psycho-Geriatrics	4	140
Paediatrics/Child Psychiatry	4	140
Total 2nd Year	**16**	**560**
Optional	5	175
3rd Year		
Medicine	4	140
Surgery	6	210
Psychiatry	4	140
Geriatrics/Psycho-Geriatrics	3	105
Public Health	3	105
Total 3rd Year	**20**	**700**
Optional/Nights	6	210
Overall Total	**65**	**2,275**

Source: **Ministere des affaires Sociales de la Sante et de la Ville, 1992.**

In accordance with Article 4 of Decree 81-306 (1981), nurse training institutions requesting recognition for the first time, and those already in existence, must lodge a submission requesting such recognition with the Director of Health and Social Services. This is forwarded to the Minister of Health together with a report stating the opinion of the Director of Health and Social Services and his rationale for this opinion. A statement must also accompany the proposal regarding how the proposal fits with the regional needs in this regard. A request from any nurse training institution already in operation must be lodged with the relevant authorities within a period of two years from the date of the Decree. Recognition is granted on the judgement of the nurse's panel of the Higher Council for paramedical professions. Withdrawal of recognition is on the same basis.

During the first academic term, nurse training institutions are required to submit to the Director of Health and Social Services an operational report which must include a statistical and academic account of the previous session (academic term), and an indication of the teaching arrangements for the current academic year. The aim of this report is to allow the Director of Health and Social Services to evaluate the match between objectives set, resources made available, and academic results achieved.

The Director of the Training school can suspend any student lacking in theoretical or practical studies during the academic year, after consultation with the Board. The Director is required to give advance notice of this, at least a fortnight before a meeting of the Board. Further, each member of the Board must be furnished with a copy of a detailed report and the student's academic record. The Director also seeks the opinion of the Board on requests from students to repeat assessments, as well as on requests for admission to training. He also seeks advice from the Board on requests from students who must repeat part of their training, to transfer to a different hospital for that purpose. In such a case, the Director is not permitted to arrange a transfer outward unless the student is guaranteed a place in another institution. Transfer requests from students may be granted only in exceptional circumstances, and only after agreement of the two Directors involved. The director must give the student reasons for the decision that is made in this regard. Cases of students finding difficulties with their studies shall be referred to the Board by the Director. The Board may suggest any specific assistance likely to solve the student's problems, but without extension of the course of study.

4.5 Disciplinary Committee

In each training school or centre a disciplinary committee is established to assist the Director with the management of student affairs. This committee is set up at the start of each academic year, when the first meeting of the Board of Studies is held. It offers judgement on disciplinary offences and acts by students that are incompatible with the safety of patients, or those that bring into question the student's personal responsibility. The committee may recommend the following sanctions:

— warning,

— reprimand

— suspension,

— expulsion.

Any such punishment is to be announced by the Director with reasons for it duly indicated. The student involved must be informed of the decision and the reasons for it. A warning may be issued by the director without her/him having to consult the committee. In such cases, students must be give prior access to their records and may request an interview with the Director and be accompanied by one person of their choice. Any student subject to such sanction must be informed of it and of the reasons for it.

Summary

While this is but a very brief and somewhat patchy overview of nurse education in France, it does give some indications of the differences and similarities between that country and others reviewed here. It would appear that there are many similarities in the curriculum content and some in the structure of the programme, with those that pertain in other countries, there are also many differences. For example, it appears that much of the regulatory functions pertaining to nurse education are conducted at a local level through the Boards of Studies. France does not have a nursing board at a national level as such, therefore much of the regulation of nursing occurs at local school of nursing level through these Boards, and at hospital level. There are also differences in who teaches nurses and what qualifications are required. Clinical nurses and nurse managers seem to feature prominently in the nurse education programmes, and it is set out above what criteria they must fulfil before they can engage in such teaching.

It is also evident that pre-registration nurse education in France is still conducted in schools of nursing within hospitals, and that there has not as yet been any substantial move to the higher education sector. Having said that, there are programmes of study at such institutes, for example there are diploma level courses that are mandatory if one wishes to become a ward sister/charge nurse. However, the extent of such links is unclear.

An Overview of the main features of Pre-Registration Nurse Education Programmes in other European countries is presented as Appendix A.

CONCLUSION

In this section, in conclusion, a reflection on the main themes of the report will be made.

A Generalist Model

A number of different curriculum models have been used in these countries, however, it would appear that there is now a tendency towards a generalist model of pre-registration nurse education. For example, it would appear that both Australia and New Zealand have by now completely adopted such an approach, and further, much of the baccalaureate pre-registration programmes in Canada follow a generalist model. Moreover, Barr and Sines (1996) report that most European countries except the United Kingdom and the Republic of Ireland, do not adopt an approach of discrete branches in nursing. The United Kingdom has so far held back from moving in the generalist model direction, however, there is some debate in the literature that such an approach should be considered. In particular, the Royal College of Nursing (1997) has advocated a generalist approach on the premise that this is a model which will enable future nurses to integrate nursing practice with other healthcare workers in order to meet the healthcare needs of a rapidly changing world. Furthermore, Barr and Sines (1996) suggests that this approach would unite the family of nursing and provide a firm foundation for post-registration specialist studies. Both Barr and Sines (1996) and the RCN express concern that recent European Union initiatives on the education and training of nurses suggest a generalist model, and that neither the Project 2000 curriculum nor the curriculum for the new pre-registration degree programmes in the UK conform to this approach. Similarly, in Canada it has been suggested that a generalist prepared nurse is the logical health professional to deliver primary health care, and this is in tandem with both national and international health policies in the developed world, for example the World Health Organisation, (1985).

Generalist models have not been without their problems however. Evidence from New Zealand and from Australia demonstrates how in many instances the general nursing component of the programme dominates even in some cases, to the complete exclusion of theory and/or clinical practice in for example, mental health nursing (Farrell and Carr, 1996; O'Brien, 1995). The difficulty here is that once registered, the generalist nurse is "qualified" to work as a first line nurse in general, mental health, children's, or learning disability nursing, this despite the foregoing. Furthermore, Barr and Sines (1996) have argued that without specialist teaching and opportunities to apply theory to clinical practice in speciality areas of nursing, generalist prepared nurses will be deficient in clinical skills. Also, that people currently cared for by specialist nurses would be cared for by nurses who have only a basic understanding of their abilities and needs.

While it would appear that the generalist route is the most popular one for the educational preparation of the nurse of the future, care is needed in constructing curricula and in monitoring its implementation. Structures need to be built into these curricula in order to ensure that the "minority" specialities of mental health, children's and learning disability nursing are not consumed and lost. Such an approach also has implications for the future nurse teacher, particularly the teacher in the clinical area. Such an individual clearly needs to have more than just a basic understanding of the former specialities now within the generalist model.

Lack of Qualifications among Nurse Teachers

That nurse teachers were poorly prepared for the transition to the higher education sector is also evident from the literature. Many were lacking in the necessary qualifications to teach in these institutions the result of which was that there was great pressure to become a graduate or to get a higher degree. In the United Kingdom at the time of the launch of Project 2000, a minority of nurse teachers were graduates, and hence when the ENB (1985) announced its requirement that all nurse teachers should become graduates, much pressure was placed on these individuals. Moreover, there was great confusion and lack of direction in regard to what type of degree to pursue. As a result it would appear that in some cases any degree that was available was chosen. It is also evident that educators in Canada were also lacking appropriate academic qualifications, however here the issue was to do with higher degrees. In Canada the majority of nurse teachers were graduates however, most community colleges required their faculty to be prepared to master's degree level, while it would appear that universities required a doctorate. Many of these latter colleges made an exception for nurse educators however and accorded them lecturer status if they had a master's degree. This was further complicated by the lack of higher degree in nursing programmes particularly in Canada. As a result, many nurse educators pursued master's and doctoral studies in subjects other than nursing, the result here being that it is unlikely that these academics will contribute as much to the development of nursing research and knowledge as would those who undertook nursing programmes at this level. Moreover, in Australia the concern was that while there were many nurse educators with master's degrees, few of these had taken a master's research degree and hence, again there is the concern that nursing knowledge will develop at an attenuated rate and slower than it might have done if higher degrees in research had been pursued. The other concern of course is that without higher degree research programmes at both master's and doctoral level, it is unlikely that nursing leadership potential will be developed, and this also is seen as a factor that will impede the overall academic and professional development of nursing.

It would appear from the foregoing that the development of a higher degree/research infrastructure in nursing is of paramount importance if nursing is going to be able to maintain academic credibility in higher education institutions. Such a level of academic qualification is also necessary if clinical practice is to develop in tandem with pre-registration and post-registration nursing programmes in higher education. Many of the problems encountered by new graduates from the programmes described in this report stemmed from an incongruence between the values of the staff in the clinical areas and those of the graduate.

Loss of Identity

One of the key issues that emerged for nurse educators in these countries immediately before and during the transition to higher education, was that of a fear of losing ones identity because of entering a different culture. This was a major theme from the interviews with nurse teachers in the Project 2000 demonstration districts in the United Kingdom, as well as for nurse teachers in Canada and Australia. Traditional nurse education in these countries had evolved from the Nightingale model, and a strong ethos of teaching and learning, and of excellence in clinical practice was common to all. Furthermore, teaching in this model was pedagogical in nature, and while there was much evidence that nurse education was moving towards more student-centred learning, this was not so in all cases. Indeed it has been suggested that one of the reasons why many nurse teachers fail to change their teaching focus in the direction of student centredness is that they cannot, as they also are products of this traditional approach to learning. Many teachers value highly these principles and certainly in hospital based schools of nursing, they were in a powerful position in regard to such education issues, and hence, often the status quo was maintained.

Higher education on the other hand, while placing some value on teaching and learning and less on clinical skills, valued most such scholarly activities as research and publishing. The high emphasis on teaching in nursing while laudable however, does not fit well with the academic model of higher education.

In particular, there was a fear among many nurse educators that the higher education colleges would take over, and that nurse educators would no longer have control over nurse education. For example, some felt that nurses should continue to teach the biological and social sciences as they are best placed to apply this to nursing. While this is a moot point, institutes of higher education almost universally require the educator to have specialist qualifications at higher degree level in the subject area they teach. Few nurse teachers fulfil these criteria for subjects other than nursing. Indeed, some of these concerns are well founded, particularly in the light of recent anecdotal evidence that historians in some UK higher education institutions, are now teaching nursing history to nursing students. Another concern in this regard was that of Professor Jill White in New Zealand, who is urging nursing to hold back from transferring from the polytechs to the university colleges. Professor White argues that such a move is pre-mature as nursing has not yet developed a strong enough research base or profile in post-graduate studies, and hence the author fears nursing will be taken over by faculties of medicine. It is arguable however that universities have much to offer nursing in this regard in that such activities as research and post-graduate education are highly valued in these colleges. Furthermore, universities can provide the resources available to develop in these activities. Perhaps another challenge to nursing is to develop clinical learning, and to work in collaboration with clinical nurses on research projects, the focus of which is clinical practice. This may lend some weight towards better academic recognition of clinical teaching and clinical skills in nursing.

Outcomes

There have been many outcome similarities in diploma and degree programmes in terms of the type of nurse that is produced. Perhaps the overriding themes from the outcome studies reviewed relate to a lack of clinical practice skills and of confidence (Elkan et al, 1993; Robertson, 1993). While there is evidence from the UK, Canada, New Zealand and

Australia that this is to some extent the case, it would also appear that this situation is short-lived. Evidence is from a number of these outcome studies that the new graduates while at the beginning are deficient in these regards, they learn quickly and are able to assimilate their superior theoretical knowledge into clinical practice. Further, estimates have been made on how long it takes these nurses to "catch up" with their traditionally prepared counterparts in clinical nursing skills, and these vary from six to twelve months. A number of initiatives have been proposed, and some are in operation, the focus of which is to gradually introduce the new graduate to professional clinical practice. These include internships, graduate nurse programmes, orientation periods, delayed registration and preceptorship. The main difficulty with these approaches across the countries studied is that in many cases such initiatives are not a required part of the pre-registration programme. Rather, they depend very much on the individual employment agency. For example, in the UK it is reported that the ENB recommends that preceptorship arrangements are in place for student's clinical placements, this is not a requirement however, and hence there is great variability in the extent to which such initiatives are used. Similarly, in Canada and Australia, many employers require that new graduates participate in a *de facto* internship, however, this does not appear to be mandatory for registration.

There is also evidence that students from the UK and Canadian pre-registration programmes are more developed in regard to self-directed and lifelong learning, and that they do not see initial registration as the final stage in their learning. However of some concern is the suggestion that graduates, despite academic studies, are still lower than the average student in regard to a number of attributes such as achievement, dominance, change and autonomy, and that they score higher in nurturance (Dyck et al., 1991). The concern that these authors express is that despite the aims of the programme (autonomy, critical thinking, decision-making and change agent), it is still possible that a near to stereotype nurse will be produced, and hence greater emphasis should be placed on entry characteristics.

While it is too early to draw conclusions regarding how long these graduates stay in nursing, and what areas of nursing they prefer to practice in, there is some preliminary evidence to suggest that a similar pattern to the early outcome studies from the UK is emerging (Milligan, 1997). These early graduates stay in nursing, particularly in areas that accord them a high degree of autonomy such as community and midwifery. Contrary to the expectations of traditionally prepared nurses, they are not fast-tracked to nursing management or education positions.

Lack of Preparation

The final theme to emerge from the review was that in many cases there was a distinct lack of preparation for the transfer to higher education. In the case of Project 2000 it emerged that in some areas nurse educators had less than six months notice in which to develop a new curriculum, while at the same time continue their commitment to the traditional programme and to other teaching commitments. Also, as has already been pointed out, many had to fit in their own undergraduate or postgraduate studies at the same time. One of the reasons for this lack of advance notice in the UK was the uncertainty of funding from the Department of Health (NAO, 1992). There was also evidence of a rushed start in some instances in Canada, where unexpectedly during the collaboration process, finance suddenly became available typically through a State grant.

The result of this sudden and unexpected funding was that the whole collaboration process was speeded up and hence staff were overworked.

There is also evidence of a lack of preparation in the clinical areas. Studies from the UK (Jowett et al., 1994), and from Australia (National Review, 1994) all suggest that staff in the clinical areas were unsure of their role in the new programme, indeed it would appear that many knew very little about the programme and its aims. Further, there was also a lack of preparation for clinical supervision of students. That these issues need to be addressed in the overall organisation and implementation of such educational change, is obvious. Despite all the preparation of the programme itself and of the teaching component, if staff in the clinical areas are ambivalent or unsure of their role or of the nature of the programme, there is the risk that all the hard work which went into the preparation of the other components of the programme will be in vain. Clearly, clinical staff need to be involved from the outset and a system of communication and information dissemination is vital. Evidence from the implementation of Project 2000 in the UK suggests that many nurse teachers did not feel a part of the process either, as they were not kept informed of developments, nor were they included in curriculum planning (Payne et al, 1991).

The above are the main themes that emerged from the literature reviewed pertaining to Australian, New Zealand, United Kingdom, and Canadian nurse education. What is perhaps most common to all was that there was a long history in each country of efforts to move nurse education forward and to bring it in par with the status and level of academic development of other health professions. Moreover, the final move to higher education often came about as a result of factors outside of the profession itself, principally, the political will that pertained at the time.

REFERENCES

Acton, L., Gough, P. and McCormak, B. (1992) The clinical nurse tutor debate. *Nursing Times* 88 (32), 38-40.

Alberta Association of Registered Nurses. (1989) Position paper on graduate education in nursing. *AARN* April, 25-26.

Allen, C. (1993) Empowerment: Taking Chances, Making Changes, in Dolan, B.(Ed) *Project 2000: Reflection and Celebration*. London: Scutari Press.

Allen, D. (1990a) Critical social theory and nursing education, in National League for Nursing. *Curriculum revolution: redefining the student teacher relationship*. New York: National League for Nursing.

Allen, D. (1990b) The curriculum revolution: radical revisioning of nursing education. *Journal of Nursing Education* 29 (7), 312-316.

Altschul, A. (1987) Why higher education for nurses? Issues and developments. *Nurse Education Today* 7, 10-16.

Altschul, A. (1983) Nursing and higher education. *International Journal of Nursing Studies* 30 (1), 123-130.

Auld, M. (1987) The need for nurse graduates in Scotland: a view from the Scottish Home and Health Department. *Nurse Education Today* 7, 30-33.

Australian Nursing Corporation Inc., (1993) *ANC Newsletter*, Number 1, December.

Battersby, D. and Hemmings, L. (1991) Clinical performance of university nursing graduates. *The Australian Journal of Advanced Nursing* 9 (1), 30-34.

Baines, C. (1992) College-university collaboration. *The Canadian Nurse* 88 (6), 17-22.

Barr, O. and Sines, D. (1996) The development of the generalist nurse within pre-registration nurse education in the UK: some points for consiedration. *Nurse Education Today* 16, 274-277.

Baumgart, A. and Kirkwood, R. (1990) Social reforms versus educational reform: University education in Canada 1919-1960. *Journal of Advanced Nursing* 15 (15), 210-216.

Beaton, J. (1990) Crisis in graduate nursing education. *The Canadian Nurse* 86 (1), 29-32.

Becker, P. (1995) Cross currents. *Research in Nursing and Health* 18, 191.

Bennett, M. (1996) The challenges of cuts to education: whither nursing education? *Collegian* 3 (4), 3-4.

Bentley, H. (1996) The need for change in nurse education: a literature review. *Nurse Education Today* 16, 131-136.

Bevis, E. and Murray, J. (1990) The essence of the curriculum revolution: emancipatory teaching. *Journal of Nursing Education* 29 (7), 326-331.

Bircumshaw, D. and Chapman, C. (1988) A follow-up of the graduates of the Cardiff Bachelor of Nursing Degree Course. *Journal of Advanced Nursing* 13, 273-279.

Burnard, P. and Morrison, P. (1992) Students' and lecturers' preferred teaching styles. *International Journal of Nursing Studies* 28 (4), 345-353..

Burnard, P. and Chapman, C. (1990) *Nurse Education: The Way Forward*. London: Scutari Press.

Burnard, P. (1986) Encountering Adults. *Senior Nurse* 4 (4), 30-31.

Burke, L. (1993) The future of the specialist nurse teacher: two different models explored. *Nurse Education Today* 13, 40-46.

Canadian Association of University Schools of Nursing. (1991) *Student and Faculty Statistical Summary for CAUSN 1984-1989*. Ottawa: CAUSN.

Carlisle, C., Kirk, S. and Luker, K. (1997) The clinical role of nurse teachers within a Project 2000 course framework. *Journal of Advanced Nursing* 25, 386-395.

Carlisle, C., Kirk, S. and Luker, K. (1996) The changes in the role of the nurse teacher following the formation of links with higher education. *Journal of Advanced Nursing* 24, 762-770.

Carlisle, C. (1991) Post-registration degrees in nursing: a time for evaluation. *Nurse Education Today* 11, 295-302.

Casey, G. (1996) The curriculum revolution and Project 2000: a critical examination. *Nurse Education Today* 16, 115-120.

Casey, N. (1990) Spanning the great divide. *Nursing Standard* 4 (24), 3.

Castledine, G. (1992) Nursing degrees: hindrance or help? *British Journal of Nursing* 1 (13), 671.

Cave, I. (1994) Nurse teachers in higher education – without clinical competence, do they have a future? *Nurse Education Today* 14, 394-399.

Cawley, S., Bopp, A., Schofer, K., Langenburg, A. and Matheis-Kraft, C. (1994) An innovative model for clinical teaching. *Nurse Educator* 19 (3), 23-25.

Chandler, J. (1991) Reforming nurse education 1 – the reorganisation of nursing knowledge. *Nurse Education Today* 11, 83-88.

Chapman, C. (1996) High Interest. *Nursing Standard* 10 (40), 51.

Charlwood, J. (1993) The Challenge of Higher Education, in Dolan, B.(Ed) *Project 2000: Reflection and Celebration*. London: Scutari Press.

Clarke, J. and Warr, J. (1995) Improved by degrees. *Nursing Times* 91 (37), 51-53.

Clay, T. (1987) *Nurses, Power and Politics*. London: Heinemann.

Clegg, C. (1992). P2000 student demands fairness. *Nursing Times* 88 (47), 12-13.

Clifford, C. (1992) The role of the nurse teacher. *Nurse Education Today* 12, 340-349.

Coburn, J. (1974) I see and am silent: A short history of nursing in Ontario – 1850-1930, in Acton, J., Goldsmith, P. and Shepherd, B. (Eds). *Women at Work*. Toronto: Canadian Women's Press.

Cowper, A. (1989) The joint appointment that works. *Midwife, Health Visitor and Community Nurse* 25 (10), 420-422.

Crotty, M. (1993) Clinical role activities of nurse teachers in Project 2000 programmes. *Journal of Advanced Nursing* 18, 460-464.

Crotty, M. and Butterworth, T. (1992) The emerging role of the nurse teacher in Project 2000 programmes in England: a literature review. *Journal of Advanced Nursing* 17, 1377-1387.

Crowther, A. (1994) Nursing's new cultural revolution. *Contemporary Nurse* 3 (4), 196.

Dahl, M. (1992) Nurses: An image change still needed. *International Nursing Review* 39 (4), 121-123.

Darbyshire, P. (1991) The American revolution. *Nursing Times* 87 (6), 57-58.

Darbyshire, P., Steward, B., Jamieson, L. and Tongue, C. (1990) New domains in Nursing. *Nursing Times* 86 (27), 73-75.

Davies, S., White, E., Riley, E., and Twinn, S. (1996) How can nurse teachers be more effective in practice settings? *Nurse Education Today* 16, 19-27.

Department of Health (1994) *Shaping a Healthier Future: A Strategy for the 1990s.* Dublin: Government Publications Stationery Office.

Department of Health (1989) *Project 2000: A Guide to Implementation.* London: HMSO.

Department of Health and Social Security (1978) *Report to the Co-ordinating Committee* (Briggs co-ordinating committee. Working group No. 2). London: HMSO.

Department of Health and Social Security (1972) *Report of the Committee on Nursing* (Briggs Report). London: HMSO.

Dewis, M, McQueen. and Grenier, F. (1993) Partnership in education: working toward the baccalaureate degree as entry to nursing practice in Canada. *Journal of Advanced Nursing* 19, 1016-1022.

Diekelman, N (1990) Nursing education: caring, dialogue and practice. *Journal of Nursing Education* 29 (7), 300-305.

Dolan, B. (1993) (Ed) *Project 2000: Reflection and Celebration.* London: Scutari Press.

Dolan, B. (1991) Power to the project? *Nursing Standard.* 5 (28), 47.

Dunn, S. (1995) CACCN and the National Review of Nursing Education. *Australian Critical Care* 8 (1), 5-8.

Dyck, S., Rae, D., Sawatzky, J. and Innes, J. (1991) Entry and exit characteristics of baccalaureate nursing students. *The Canadian Journal of Nursing Research* 23 (1), 27-40.

Elkan, R., Hillman, R. and Robinson, J. (1993) *The Implementation of Project 2000 in a District Health Authority: The Effect on Nursing service.* (Second Interim Report) University of Nottingham: Department of Nursing and Midwifery Studies.

Elzubier, M. and Sherman, M. (1995) Nursing skills and practice. *British Journal of Nursing* 4 (18), 1087-1092.

English National Board (1996) *Project 2000: Perceptions of the philosophy and practice of nursing.* London: ENB.

English National Board (1989) *Project 2000: A new preparation for practice.* London: ENB.

English National Board (1985) *Professional education/training courses: consultation paper.* London: ENB.

Farrell, G. and Carr, J. (1996) Who cares for the mentally ill? Theory and practice hours with a mental illness' focus in nursing curricula in Australian universities. *Australian and New Zealand Journal of Mental Health Nursing* 5, 77-83.

Field, P. (1989) Implementing change in nursing education. *Nurse Education Today* 9, 290-299.

Fitzpatrick, J., While, A. and Robinson, J. (1993) The relationship between nursing and higher education. *Journal of Advanced Nursing* 18, 1488-1497.

Forsyth, S. (1995) Historical Continuities and constraints in the professionalization of nursing. *Nursing Inquiry* 2, 164-171.

French, S. (1992) Reform in higher education for nurses: comparative comments from Canada. *Contemporary Nurse* 1 (2), 54-67.

Furner, B. (1996) Polytechnics fail to serve nursing. *Kai Tiaki: Nursing New Zealand* 2 (2), 3-4.

Gallagher, P. (1995) An educator looks in. *Kai Tiaki: Nursing New Zealand* 1 (4), 17.

Gibbon, J. and Mathewson, M. (1947) *Three Centuries of Canadian Nursing.* Toronto: Macmillan.

Gibbs, I. and Rush, B. (1987) Higher education: the coping stone of nursing education? *Journal of Advanced Nursing* 12, 659-669.

Glasper, P. and O'Connor, S. (1996) Nursing should be an all graduate profession. *British Journal of Nursing* 5 (1), 5.

Goldenberg, D., Gerhard, W., McFadden, A. and Johnston, E. (1995) Collaboration in nursing education. *The Canadian Nurse* 91 (1), 21-25.

Gott, M. (1984) *Learning Nursing.* London: RCN.

Gough, P., Maslin-Prothero, S. and Masterson, A. (1993) A reflection on Issues for Practice, in Dolan, B.(Ed) *Project 2000: Reflection and Celebration*. London: Scutari Press.

Grant, E., Ives, G., Raybould, J. and O'Shea, M. (1996) Clinical nurses as teachers of nursing students. *Australian Journal of Advanced Nursing* 14 (2), 24-30.

Grant, N. (1995) Vocation or profession? *The Canadian Nurse* 91 (6), 8.

Hanson, K.S. (1989) The emergence of liberal education in nursing education 1893-1923. *Journal of Professional Nursing* 5 (2), 83-91.

Happell, B. (1996) Tertiary psychiatric nursing graduates: something different or more of the same? *Australian and New Zealand Journal of Mental Health Nursing* 5, 112-119.

Hart, G. and Rotem, A. (1994) The best and the worst: students experiences of clinical education *The Australian Journal of Advanced Nursing* 11 (3), 26-33.

Hart, G. (1985) College based education: background and bugs. *The Australian Nurses Journal* 15 (4), 46-48.

Harvey, J. (1988) Life's not easy when you're first through a course, but... *The Australian Journal of Advanced Nursing* 5 (4), 19-21.

Harloe, L., Greenway, M., Fowle, T., Hayes, K., Pendall, D., Stewart, C., Squires, L., Bond, M. and White, K. (1995) Generating ideas for research: An Australian Research Experience. *Gastroenterology Nursing* 18 (4), 138-141.

Hayward, J. (1982) Universities and nurse education. *Journal of Advanced Nursing* 7, 371-377.

Hempel, P. (1990) Identification of the need for nursing education. *AARN* 46 (10), 29.

Henry, C. and Pashley, G. (1989) Vital links. *Nursing Times* 85 (27), 70-71.

Hickey, G. (1996) The challenge of change in nurse education: traditionally trained nurses' perceptions of Project 2000. *Nurse Education Today* 16, 389-396.

Hill, E. and Kirkwood, R. (1991) *Breaking down the walls: Nursing Science at Queens University*. Kingston: Brown and Martin.

Hiscott, R. (1995) Changes in the school-to-work transition for Canadian nursing Program Graduates. *Canadian Journal of Nursing Research* 27 (4), 151-163.

Horsburgh, M. (1990/91) Polytech by degrees. *New Zealand Nursing Journal* 83 (11), 27.

Horsburgh, M. (1989) Graduate nurses' adjustment to initial employment: natural field work. *Journal of Advanced Nursing* 14, 610-617.

Horsburgh, M., Baker, H., Hartford, V., Jones, M., Rhodes, E. and Smythe, L. (1989) Achievement and learning processes in nursing students. *Nursing Praxis in New Zealand* 4 (3), 20-26.

Howard, J. and Brooking, J. (1987) The career paths of nursing graduates from Chelsea College, University of London. *International Nursing Studies* 24 (3), 181-189.

Hudson, S. (1996) Education cuts short sighted. *Australian Nursing Journal* 4 (2), 15.

Hughes, M. (1998) Personal Communication- Former Senior Lecturer in Nursing, Buckinghamshire College, Brunel University.

Ives, G. and Rowley, G. (1990) A clinical learning milieu: nurse clinicians attitudes to tertiary education and teaching. *The Australian Journal of Advanced Nursing* 7 (4), 29-35.

Jasper, M. (1996) The first year as a staff nurse: the experiences of a first cohort of project 2000 nurses in a demonstration district. *Journal of Advanced Nursing* 24, 779-790.

Jones, C. (1996) The client in 4A. *Contemporary Nurse* 5 (3), 134.

Jones, J. (1985) A study of nurse tutors' conceptualisations of their ward teaching role. *Journal of Advanced Nursing* 10, 349-360.

Jowett, S., Walton, I. and Payne, S. (1994) *Challenges and Change in Nurse Education- A Study of the Implementation of Project 2000*. Slough: National Foundation for Educational Research.

Kaur, M. Gallagher, F. (1995) Get to know the nurses of the future. *The Queensland Nurse* Sept/Oct, 14-17.

Kemp, J. (1988) Graduates in nursing: a report of a longitudinal study at the University of Hull. *Journal of Advanced Nursing* 13, 281-287.

Kershaw, B. (1996) An open letter. *Nursing Standard* 10 (27), 55.

Kershaw, B. (1990) Clinical Credibility and nurse teachers. *Nursing Standard* 4 (51), 46-47.

King Edward's Hospital Fund for London. (1984) *Joint clinical appointments in nursing*. London: King's Fund.

King, K. (1970) The development of university nursing education, in Innes, M. (Ed). *Nursing Education in a Changing Society*. Toronto: Toronto University Press.

Kirk, S,. Carlisle, C. and Luker, K. (1997) The implications of Project 2000 and the formation of links with higher education for the professional and academic needs of nurse teachers in the United Kingdom. *Journal of Advanced Nursing* 26, 1036-1044.

Knowles, M. (1980) *The Modern Practice of Adult Education*. 2nd Edn. Chicago: Follett.

Lathlean, J. (1992) The contribution of lecturer practitioners to theory and practice in nursing. *Journal of Clinical Nursing* 1, 237-242.

Lathlean, J. (1987) Prepared Transition. *Nursing Times* 83 (37), 42-47.

Leonard, A. and Jowett, S. (1990) *Charting the Course: A Study of the Six ENB Pilot Schemes in Pre-registration Nurse Education* (Research Paper No 1). Slough: National Foundation for Educational Research.

Logan, W. (1987) Is education for a nursing elite? Some highlights in nursing education in Europe and North America. *Nurse Education Today* 7, 5-9.

Lowery, B. J. (1991) Resources to maintaining the academic culture. *Journal of Professional Nursing* 7 (3), 177-183.

Luker, K. (1984) Reading nursing: the burden of being different. *International Journal of Nursing Studies* 21 (1), 1-7.

Lumby, J. (1989) Preparation for Practice, in, Gray, G., and Pratt, R. (Eds). *Issues in Australian Nursing*. Melbourne: Churchill Livingstone.

MacGuire, J. (1991) Nurses with degrees in the United Kingdom: careers and contributions and challenges. *Journal of Advanced Nursing* 16, 625-627.

MacGuire, J. and Sparks, S. (1970) The nurse graduate in the United Kingdom: patterns of qualification. *International Nursing Review* 17, 350-372.

Madjar, I. (1995) Nursing and the academe: advance or retreat? *Nursing Inquiry* 2, 129-130.

Marquis, B., Lillibridge, J. and Madison, J. (1993) Problems and progress as Australia adopts the Bachelor's degree as the only entry to practice. *Nursing Outlook* 41 (3), 135-140.

Marsh, N. (1976) Summary report of a study of the career patterns of dipolmates/graduates of the undergraduate nursing course in the University of Manchester, England. *Journal of Advanced Nursing* 1, 539-542.

Mason, J. (1991a) Nurses in the education industry. Conference proceedings: Power and Politics in the Health Professions. Northern territory, Darwin.

Mason, J. (1991b) Project 2000: a critical review. *Nursing Practice* 4 (3), 2-5.

Mauksch, I. and Styles, M. (1982) From Nurse-to-Nurse Educator: The Socialisation of Nurses into the Faculty Role. in, Henderson, M.S. (Ed). *Recent Advances in Nursing: Nursing Education*. Edinburgh: Churchill Livingstone.

McFarlane, Baroness. (1987) The role of nurse graduates in the health service in the year 2000. *Nurse Education Today* 7, 38-41.

Melchior-MacDougall, F. (1992) Specialisation in nursing: it's history and its future. *AARN* 48 (1), 7-8.

Milligan, F. (1997) The Move towards pre-registration nursing degree programmes in the UK: A literature review- Conference Summary. Un published conference proceedings. NET 97 Conference.

Ministere des Affaires Sociales de la Sante et de la Ville (Undated). Recueil des Principaux Textes Relatifs a la Formation et a L'Exercise de la Profession D'Infirmier.

Ministry of Health. (1947) *The Recruitment and Training of Nurses* (Wood Report). London: HMSO.

Montague, S. and Herbert, R. (1982) Career paths of graduates of a degree-linked nursing course. *Journal of Advanced Nursing* 7, 359-370.

Naish, J. (1996) Scarce resources. *Nursing Times* 92 (32), 32-33.

Naish, J. (1993) Power, Politics and Peril, in Dolan, B.(Ed) *Project 2000: Reflection and Celebration*. London: Scutari Press.

Naish, J. (1990) Project 2000 anger. *Nursing Standard* 4 (26), 24.

National Audit Office. (1992) *Nursing Education: Implementation of Project 2000 in England. Report of the Comptroller and Auditor General.* London:HMSO.

National Review (1994) *Nursing Education in Australian Universities. Report of the National Review of Nurse Education in The Higher Education Sector- 1994 and beyond.* Canberra: Australian Government Publishing Service.

Neill, J. and Barclay, L. (1989) Sociodemographic characteristics of nursing students in higher education. *The Australian Journal of Advanced Nursing* 7 (1), 4-11.

Newton, L. (1981) In defence of the traditional nurse. *Nursing Outlook* 29, 348-354.

Nurse Education Today (1987) The time for change (Editorial). *Nurse Education Today* 7, 47-48.

Nurses Association of New Brunswick (1994) NANB welcomes change in entry point. *Info Nursing* 26 (1), 4.

Nursing Standard (1996) Poverty is the real issue. *Nursing Standard* 10 (40), 50.

Nursing Times (1996) Wishful thinking. *Nursing Times* 92 (32), 31-32.

O'Brien, A. (1995) Measuring graduate attitudes to educational preparation for practice in mental health nursing. *Australian and New Zealand Journal of Mental Health Nursing* 4, 132-142.

O'Connor, T. (1996) Whats the future for nursing education? *Kai Tiaki: Nursing New Zealand* 2 (7), 28-29.

Orr, J. (1987) Why shouldn't we be clever? *Nursing Times* 83 (35), 24.

Owen, G. (1988) For better, for worse: nursing in higher education. *Journal of Advanced Nursing* 13 (3), 13.

Parker, T. and Carlisle, C. (1996) Project 2000 students' perceptions of their training. *Journal of Advanced Nursing* 24, 771-778.

Payne, S., Jowett, S. and Walton, I. (1991) *Nurse Teachers in Project 2000: The Experience of Planning and Initial Implementation*. Slough: National Foundation for Educational Research.

Pelletier, D., Duffield, C., Gallagher, R., Soars, L., Donoghue, J. and Adams, A. (1994) The effects of graduate nurse education on clinical practice and career paths: a pilot study. *Nurse Education Today*14, 314-321.

Prebble, K. and McDonald, B. (1997) Adaptation to mental health setting: The lived experience of comprehensive nurse graduates. *Australian and New Zealand Journal of Mental Health Nursing* 6, 30-36.

Prew, C. (1989) Thoughts on a new curriculum. *Nursing Times* 85 (10), 70-71.

Reid, N., Nellis, P. and Boore, J. (1987) Graduate nurses in Northern Ireland: their career paths, aspirations and problems. *International Journal of Nursing Studies* 24 (3), 215-225.

Reid, N. (1986) Recent manpower trends in Northern Ireland. *International Journal of Nursing Studies* 23, 199-210.

Rhead, M. and Strange, F. (1996) Nursing lecturer/practitioners: can lecturer/practitioners be music to our ears? *Journal of Advanced Nursing* 24, 1265-1272.

Robinson, J. (1993) All Change: Project 2000's Greatest Challenge, in Dolan, B.(Ed) *Project 2000: Reflection and Celebration*. London: Scutari Press.

Robinson, J. (1991) Project 2000: the role of resistance in the process of professional growth. *Journal of Advanced Nursing* 16, 820-824.

Ross, E. (1995) Letter From Canada. *Nursing Times* 91 (25), 77.

Royal College of Nursing (1997) The future of nurse education. *Nursing Standard* 11 (34). 22-24.

Royal College of Nursing (1994) *Must it be so hard? Hardship amongst nursing students*. London: RCN.

Royal College of Nursing (1985) *The Education of Nurses: A New Dispensation* (Judge Report). London: RCN.

Royal College of Nursing (1964) *A reform of Nurse Education* (Platt Report). London: RCN.

Royal College of Nursing (1943) *Nursing Reconstruction Committee* (Horder Report). London: RCN.

Royal College of Nursing, Australia (1996) Nurse education to improve. *Collegian* 3 (1), 11-13.

Rundell, S. (1990) Is stripe-itis curable? *Nursing Times* 86 (42). 23.

Russell, L. (1992) *In the vanguard: nursing in Australia*. New South Wales: NSW College of Nursing.

Russell, L. (1990) *From Nightingale to now: Nurse education in Australia*. Sydney: Harcourt Brace Jovanovich.

Russell, R. (1988) Nursing education: a time for change 1960-1980. *The Australian Journal of Advanced Nursing* 5 (4), 36-37.

Sax, S. (1978). *Nurse education and training. Report of the Committee of Inquiry into nurse education and training to the tertiary education commission.* Canberra: TEC.

Scott-Wright, M., Gilmore, M. and Tierney, A. (1979) The nurse/graduate in nursing: preliminary findings of a follow-up study of former students of the university of Edinburgh degree/nursing programme. *International Journal of Nursing Studies* 16, 205-214.

Sherrard, I. (1995) NZQA: Where do nurses and midwives stand? *Kai Tiaki: Nursing New Zealand* 1 (1) (Nursing Education) 1-2.

Shorten, D. and McMurray, A. (1991) Nursing education in Australia: recent developments. *AARN* 48 (7), 38.

Simard, L. (1992) *A Saskatchewan vision for health: A framework for change*. Regina, SK: Saskatchewan Health.

Simons, W. (1984) Towards integration. *Senior Nurse* 1 (28): 14-16.

Simpson, I. (1979) *From student to nurse*. Cambridge: Cambridge University Press.

Sinclair, H. (1987) Graduate nurses in the United Kingdom: myth and reality. *Nurse Education Today* 7, 24-29.

Sinclair, H. (1984) The careers of nurse graduates. *Nursing Times* (Occasional Papers), 56-59.

Slevin, E. (1995) Student nurses' attitudes towards people with learning disabilities. *British Journal of Nursing* 4 (13), 761-766.

Sloper, B. (1994) Balancing the books. *Nursing Times* 90 (12), 58.

Smadu, M. (1995) The beginning graduate nurse in Saskatchewan. *Concern* 24 (4), 14-17.

Smith, F. (1982) *Florence Nightingale: Her Reputation and Power*. Melbourne: Croom Helm.

Snell, J. (1995) It's tough at the bottom. *Nursing Times* 91 (43), 55-58.

South Australia Health Commission. (1986) *Report of the Nurse Education Monitoring Committee*. Adelaide: SAHC.

Spence, D. (1994) The curriculum revolution: can educational reform take place without reform in practice? *Journal of Advanced Nursing* 19, 187-193.

Stodart, K. (1990/91) Graduation Blues. *New Zealand Nursing Journal* 83 (11), 28.

Taylor, A., Small, D., White, J., Hall, P. and Fenwick, P. (1981) *An Evaluation of Nursing Courses in Technical Institutes*. Wellington: Department of Education.

Thomas, B., Arseneault, J., Cote, E. and Stanton, S. (1992) Accreditation of university nursing courses in Canada. *The Canadian Journal of Nursing Research* 24 (2), 33-48.

Townsend, J. (1991) Academic nurse or n'academic: An identity crisis for nurse academics. Conference proceedings. NSW College of Nursing, 13th September.

UKCC (1987) *Project 2000. The Final Proposals.* (Project paper 9) London: UKCC.

UKCC (1986) *Project 2000: A New Preparation for Practice.* London: UKCC.

Vaughan, J. (1990) Student nurse attitudes to teaching and learning methods. *Journal of Advanced Nursing* 15, 925-933.

Wainwright, P. (1996) The immorality of pre-registration nurse education: A personal Perspective. *Nursing Ethics* 3 (1), 73-77.

Walker, C. (1979) *The newly qualified staff nurse's perception of the transition from student to trained nurse.* Un published MSc Thesis, University of Manchester, England.

Wall, K. (1991) Schooling the family. *The Canadian Nurse* 7 (11), 20-21.

Watson, J. (1994) Guest Editorial. *Nursing Praxis in New Zealand* 9 (1), 2-5.

Wells-Jansz, D. (1996) Survival of the richest. *Nursing Standard* 10 (15), 52.

Wenban, P. (1985) One school of thought. *Senior Nurse* 2 (8), 8-9.

While, A., Roberts, J. and Fitzpatrick, J. (1995) *A Comparative Study of Outcomes of Pre-registration Nurse Education Programmes.* London: ENB.

White Paper (1989) *Review of the NHS- Working for Patients.* London: HMSO.

Williams, G. (1992). Nursing education in new Zealand. *International Nursing Review* 39 (1), 21-22.

Willis, J. The threat of student loans. *Nursing Times* 92 (31), 62-63.

Wilson. K. (1996) What price nursing education? *Kai Tiaki: Nursing New Zealand* 2 (1), 26-27.

Wong, J. and Wong, S. (1987) Towards effective clinical teaching in nursing. *Journal of Advanced Nursing* 12, 505-513.

Wood, M. (1996) Education for the future. *Registered Nurse Journal* August/September, 37-38.

Wood, P. (1990) *Nursing: Progress through partnership.* Canberra: Commonwealth Department of Community Services and Health.

World Health Organisation (1994) *Partners for mental health: the contribution of professionals and non-professionals to mental health.* Geneva: WHO.

World Health Organisation (1985) *Targets for Health for All by the Year 2000.* Geneva: WHO.

Wright, C. (1988) Student participation in nursing programmes: a study of their social composition since the transfer to colleges of advanced education. *Higher Education Research and Development* 7 (2), 153-162.

Yuill, S. (1995) Get beyond education debate. *The Canadian Nurse* 91 (6), 7.

APPENDIX

1. Summary Table on Current Education and Training of Nurses Responsible for General Care in the European Union.

(II. CURRENT SITUATION (1-1-96)).

A:	GENERAL INFORMATION	NETHERLANDS		SWEDEN	LUXEMBOURG
I.	Legislative framework	Diploma HBO - Verpleegkundige (nurse) (HBO = Higher Vocational Education)	Diploma A - Verpleegkundige (nurse)	Sjuksköterskeamen/ka (nurse's) diploma (univ)	State nurse's diploma*
1.1 1.2	Diploma/qualification Are there laws and/or regulations on education and training?	at national level	at national level	at national level	at national level
1.3	Supervisory authority for nurses' education and training	Ministry of Education, Cultural Affairs and Science	Ministry of Health, Welfare and Sport	Ministry of Education/National Agency for Higher Education	Ministry of Education and Vocational Training
II. 2.1 2.2 2.3.	Training establishments Number of institutions Where based Level at which diploma recognized	19 other: 19	46 hospitals: 46	29 colleges University Diploma in Nursing corresponding with Bachelor Degree level	1 from 11.1.1995 technical lycée technical secondary education
III. 3.1	Admission requirements Access to nurse's education and training age: previous schooling: qualification: entrance exam:	17 12 or 13 Years lower or higher general secondary education depending on which training no		no limit 12 years university entrance requirements = completion secondary education yes (optional and complementary entrance examinations e.g. theoretical tests to improve grades from secondary school)	17 11 years 11th year of technical secondary education no
3.2	Access to university age: previous schooling: qualification: entrance exam:	18 14 years pre-university education no		12 years	19 12 years baccalauréat no
3.3	Is there a numerus clausus for nurses? according to what criteria?	no		yes, set by the local authorities according to expected needs in the labour market	no no

* In Luxembourg there is a graduate nurse's diploma. Various European training programmes are recognized under this diploma.

A:	GENERAL INFORMATION	NETHERLANDS		SWEDEN	LUXEMBOURG
IV.	System for monitoring the quality of education and training				
4.1	Is there a system for monitoring the quality of education and training?	no		yes	yes
4.2	How does this work? How often? according to what criteria?	visit of the training establishment once every 5 years	no	National Agency for Higher Education inspections and collection of data one report per year	a government commissioner chairs the national examination committee
B.	SPECIFIC INFORMATION				
I. 1.1	Legislative framework Diploma/qualification	Diploma HBO - Verpleegkundige	Diploma A - Verpleegkundige	Sjusköterskeamen/ka (nurse's) diploma (univ)	State nurses's diploma
II. 2.1	Admission requirements age		17		17
	previous schooling:	13 years	12 years	12 years	11 years
	qualification:	higher general secondary education or intermediate vocational education	lower general secondary education or lower vocational education	same conditions as for university	11th year of technical secondary education
	entrance exam:	no entrance exam	no extrance exam	yes	no
III. 3.1	Education and training Duration				
	years:	4 years	3 years + 10 months	3 years	3 years
	months:			30 months	
	weeks:	168 weeks	44 weeks of 30 h = 1320 h/132.5 weeks of 36 h = 4770 h	120 weeks	
	hours:	6 720 hours	6 090 hours	4 800 hours	4 600 h
	other:			120 points, 1 point = 1 week	1 h = 50 min

138

B:	SPECIFIC INFORMATION	NETHERLANDS	SWEDEN	LUXEMBOURG
3.2 a)	**Course** Total number of hours	6 720 hours	4 800 h	4 600 h
b)	Theoretical/technical training • total number of hours	3 897 hours	2 400 h	min 1 600 h
	• how subdivided			
	— nursing	1 344 hours	1 400 h	703 h
	— basic science	2 553 hours (basic science and social science)	1 000 h	927 h
	— social sciences			
c)	Clinical training • total number of hours	2 823 hours	2 400 h	min. 3 000 h
	• how subdivided	differs per training centre		
	— general medicine		600 h	min. 800 h
	— general surgery		600 h	min. 800 h
	— child care and paediatrics		40 h	min. 100 h
	— maternity care		40 h	min. 120 h
	— mental health/psychiatry		320 h	min. 200 h
	— care of the elderly		400 h	min. 120 h
	— home care		400 h	min. 860 h
	— Other			courses in intensive care, medical scanning, operating theatre, accident and emergency
3.3	Subjects not listed in the annex	Informatics, Economic Ethics related to Health care	Informatics, Economic Ethics related to Health care	
3.4	Is education and training identical in all establishments?	no	no, as establishments have some freedom regarding courses	yes, broadly speaking
IV. 4.1	**Remuneration** Remuneration for trainees — from whom?	yes Ministry of Education, Culture and Science, / the employer	no	yes, up to September 1995 the employer, reimbursed by the Ministry of Health, LFR 5 000 per month in 1st yr, LFR 7 000 in 2nd yr and LFR 9 000 in 3rd yr
	— how much?	HFL 425 per month / HFL 2 200 per month during clinical training		
	— for which courses?	whole course		
4.2	Do training establishments subsidise places where students undergo clinical training?	no	yes	no

B:	SPECIFIC INFORMATION	NETHERLANDS		SWEDEN	LUXEMBOURG
V.	Instructors				
5.1	Level of qualification required to run an establishment		No regulation	Nurse with preferably Ph D	graduate nurse or doctor
5.2	Do those running establishments have to be qualified nurses?		no	no	no
5.3	Qualification required for instructors who are nurses?	educational competence and a master in nursing	educational competence	junior: R.N., master's degree senior lecturer or professor: R.N., Ph D	graduate nurse
5.4	Is there a set student/instructor ratio?	Balance between the both	not more than 25 students per instructor	no	yes, no less than 15 students per instructor

140

A.	GENERAL INFORMATION	UNITED KINGDOM	FINLAND
I.			
1.1.	Legislative framework Diploma/qualification	State Registered Nurse, Registered General Nurse, Registered Nurse	Sairaanhoitaja/sjukskötare (diploma in nursing)
1.2.	Are there laws and/or regulations on education and training?	at national level	at national level
1.3.	Supervisory authorities	United Kingdom Central Council for Nursing, Midwifery and Health Visiting	Ministry of Education and National Board of Education
II.			
2.1.	Training establishments Number of institutions	74	36
2.2.	Where based	universities / hospitals / other (linked to univ.) E* 50% W: 66% S: 83% NI:17% 0 0 0 0 50% 33% 17% 83%	college
2.3.	Level at which diploma recognised	Academic level: BA/BSc (10%) or diploma of higher education (90%) Professional qualification (R.N.) is the same for both	Bachelor in nursing (Ammattikorkeakoulu=polytechnic) Non university higher education qualification
III.			
3.2.	Admission requirements Access to nurse's education and training age:	17½ min.; no upper limit	17, no upper limit
	previous schooling: qualification:	not applicable in UK 5 GCSE passes (taken at 16)	12 years certificate of upper secondary education
	entrance exam:	yes, the UKCC's 'DC test' for applicants who do not have 5 GCSE passes	yes, written exam, psychological tests, interview
3.1.	Access to university age:	no age requirement	
	previous schooling: qualification:	not fixed, usually 12-13 years 2 passes at higher level of school leaving certificate (taken at 18)	
	entrance exam:	varies from university to university	
3.3.	Is there a numerus clausus for nurses?	yes, health care providers determine number of nurses required 3-5 years ahead;	yes, set by the Ministry of Education on the basis of an assessment of labour market needs
	according to what criteria?	—determination of number of training places required each year —determination of number of funded training places in each region	
IV.	System for monitoring the quality of education and training		
4.1.	Is there a system for monitoring the quality of education and training?	yes, each National Board has its own system for monitoring quality	yes, National council of quality assessment (ammattikorkeakoulu). National Board of Education (other establishments) and the establishments themselves.
4.2.	How does this work? how often? according to what criteria?	parallel monitoring systems – professional: by UKCC; educational; by 'Higher Education Quality Council' regular review of programmes and teachers, courses, etc. major reviews every 5 years, lesser reviews every year	Ministry of Education and National Board of Education, through internal and external evaluation, performance agreements once a year, other evaluations irregularly.

*E=England; W=Wales; S=Scotland; NI=Northern Ireland.

B.	SPECIFIC INFORMATION	UNITED KINGDOM		FINLAND	
		DEGREE	DIPLOMA	Health care institute	Ammattikorkeakoulu
I.					
1.1.	Legislative framework Diploma/qualification				
II.					
2.1.	Admission requirements				
	age:	no age limit	no age limit	17	17
	previous schooling:	12 years	10 years	12 years	12 years
	qualification:	2 passes at Advanced level school leaving certificate (taken at 18)	5 GCSE passes (taken at 16)	certificate of upper secondary education	certificate of upper secondary education
	entrance exam:	yes	yes	yes	yes
III.					
3.1.	Education and training Duration: years:	3 or 4 years	3 years	$3\frac{1}{2}$ years	$3\frac{1}{2}$ years
	months:	at least 36	36	36	
	weeks:	at least 135	135	133	
	hours:	at least 4 600	4 600	4 655 hours	
	other:		credits for academic part	1h theory=45 min; 1h clinical=60 min.	140 credits (1 credit=40 hours)
3.2.	Course				
(a)	Total number of hours	4 600 hours	4 600 hours	4 655 h	5 600 h
(b)	Theoretical/technical training • total number of hours	variable	variable	2 682 h	3 600 h
	• how subdivided —nursing —basic science —social sciences				
(c)	Clinical training • total number of hours	variable	variable	1 973	2 000
	• how subdivided				variable
	—general medicine			748	
	—general surgery			364	
	—child care and paediatrics			122	
	—maternity care			105	
	—mental health/psychiatry			108	
	—care of the elderly			105	
	—home care			70	
3.3.	Subjects not listed in the annex	varies from institution to institution	varies from institution to institution	maths, physics, PE, sport, research studies, environmental health, languages: English, Swedish, Finnish	philosophy, statistics languages: English, Swedish, Finnish
3.4.	Is education and training identical in all establishments	yes	yes	yes	no

142

B.	SPECIFIC INFORMATION	UNITED KINGDOM		FINLAND	
		DEGREE	DIPLOMA	Health care institute	Ammattikorkeakoulu
IV.	Remuneration				
4.1	Remuneration for trainees —from whom? —how much? —for which coures?	Department of Education	yes Department of Health	no	no
4.2	Do training establishments subsidise places where students undergo clinical training?	under discussion		yes	yes
V.	Instructors				
5.1	Level of qualification required to run an establishment	in universities, the head of the programme must be a nurse	in colleges, the head of the establishment must be a nurse	Masters degree in Health Care including teacher training plus at least 3 years' experience as a teacher of nursing	
5.2	Do those running establishments have to be qualified nurses?			yes	
5.3	Qualification required for instructors who are nurses?	degree/doctorate	additional training as nurse teacher	Qualified Teacher of Nursing or M.Sc. in Health Care Sciences, minimum of two years' work experience	
5.4	Is there a set student/instructor ratio?	yes, up to 1994	yes, up to 1994	no	

143

	GENERAL INFORMATION	BELGIUM	GERMANY	AUSTRIA
A.				
I.	Legislative framework			
1.1.	Diploma/qualification	Graduate nurse's diploma, Hospital nurse's certificate	Krankenschwester/pfleger (nurse)	Krankenschwester/pfleger (nurse)
1.2.	Are there laws and/or regulations on education and training?	at national level / at regional level	at national level	at national level
1.3.	Supervisory authority for nurses' education and training	Ministry of Education, Research and Training, Ministry of Culture and Social Affairs, Council for Higher Paramedical Education	Health Ministry of Länder or Ministry of Culture	Ministry of Health and Consumer Protection, bodies responsible for health in the Länder, professional organisations
II.	Training establishments			
2.1.	Number of institutions	26 institutions (19 train for certificate, 20 for graduate diploma)	800	59
2.2.	Where based	university/schools/institutes	hospital	hospital
2.3.	Level at which diploma recognised	short, full-time higher paramedical education course (graduate diploma) complementary secondary professional education (certificate)	qualified vocational training	
III.	Admission requirements			
3.1.	Access to nurse's education and training	higher nursing training		
	training age:	no age requirement	17	16 min.—35 max.
	previous schooling:	12 years	10 years	10 years
	qualification:	secondary school certificate	'mittlere Reife'	'mittlere Reife'
	entrance exam:	no	no	yes
3.2.	Access to university			
	age:	no age requirement	no requirement	18
	previous schooling	12 years	13 years	12 years
	qualification:	secondary school certificate	'Abitur'	'Reifeprüfung'
	entrance exam:	in some faculties in the form of a written test	no	no
3.3.	Is there a numerus clausus for nurses? according to what criteria?	no	no	yes, the schools decide according to the number of places available and the demand for nurses
IV.	System for monitoring the quality of education and training			
4.1.	Is there a system for monitoring the quality of education and training?	yes	yes	yes, by the Land authorities (Landeshauptmann)
4.2.	How does this work? how often? according to what criteria?	system little used, visit by inspector 1 or 2 times a year	local or regional administration	Land administration continuous monitoring and presence at examination at least twice a year.

144

B. SPECIFIC INFORMATON	BELGIUM		GERMANY	AUSTRIA
	Graduate Nurse (diploma)	Hospital Nurse (certificate)	Krankenschwester/Pfleger	Krankenschwester/Pfleger
I. 1.1. Leg./reg. framework Diploma/qualification				
II. 2.1. Admission requirements age: Previous schooling qualifications	no age limit 12 years secondary school certificate or examining board	no age limit secondary vocational school certificate or examining board	17 10 years 'mittlere Reife'	min. 16, max. 35 10 years 'mittlere Reife'
entrance examination:	no	no	no	aptitude test which varies from one Land to another
III. 3.1. Education and training Duration: years:	3 years	3 years	3 years	3 years
months: weeks: hours:	30 weeks (besides assessment) 3 540 hours (1h=50 min.)	40 weeks with assessment 4 320 hours (1h=50 min)	4 600	5 200
3.2. Course (a) Total number of hours	3 540 h	4 320 h	4 600 h	5 200 h
(b) Theoretical/technical training • total number of hours	1 440 h	2 080 h		
• how subdivided —nursing —basic sciences —social sciences	720 h 720 h	1 160 h	500 h 1 000-1 200 h	26 % 74 %
(c) Clinical training • total number of hours	1 800 h	2 240 h	2 400-3 600 h	2 800 h
• how subdivided —general medicine —general surgery —child care and paediatrics —maternity care —mental health, psychiatry —care of the elderly —home care —other	min. 280 h min. 280 h min. 120 h min. 40 h min. 80 h 80-120 h min. 80 h 500 h	520 h 520 h 160 h 160 h 160 h 240 h 80 h	900 h 750 h 77-231 h 350 h 150-231 h included in general medicine 150-231 h 385 h	600 h 600 h 400 h 160 h
3.3. Subjects not listed in annex	Theory: schools add subjects according to their specialisation Clinical: operating theatre, accident and emergency, intensive care	schools may add subjects according to their specific needs	basic teaching in rehabilitation language and literature	English, musical and physical education, psychosomatics
3.4. Is education and training identical in all establishments?	no, the head of the establishment is free to take initiative on course	no, the head of the establishment is free to take initiative on course	no*	yes

*Training requirements (subjects and number of hours) are set at federal level, but curricula are set at regional level and, where no such standards exist, autonomously by nurses' training colleges.

145

B.	SPECIFIC INFORMATON	BELGIUM		GERMANY	AUSTRIA
IV. 4.1	Remuneration Remuneration for trainees —for whom? —how much? —for which courses?	no		yes training organisation DM 1 200 - 1 500 all	yes training organisation varies from one Land to another for the theoretical and practical part in the form of monthly pocket money
4.2	Do training establishments subsidise places where students undergo clinical training?	no		no	no
V. 5.1	Instructors Level of qualification required to run an establishment	required level: minimum degree required field: medical doctor or a counsellor having the title being associated	no information	specialised treacher training	specialised and teacher training
5.2	Do those running establishments have to be qualified nurses?	no	no	yes	
5.3	Qualification required for instructors who are nurses?	*teaching qualification and at least one year's professional experience	*teaching qualification	professional experience as a nurse and teacher training	three years' professional experience as a nurse and teaching proficiency
5.4	Is there a set student/instructor ratio?	no, an overall budget is distributed by the head of the establishment	no, an overall budget is distributed by the head of the establishment	no	yes; —theory: 1 teacher for every 15 students —clinical: the number of students cannot be more than 150% of the number of qualified nurses in the hospital

*Training requirements (subjects and number of hours) are set at federal level, but curricula are set at regional level and, where no such standards exist, autonomously by nurses' training colleges.

A. GENERAL INFORMATION	DENMARK	SPAIN	FRANCE
I. 1.1 Legislative framework Diploma/qualification	Sygeplejerske (nurse's) diploma	Titulo de Diplomado Universitario de Enfermeria (university nursing diploma)	State nurse's diploma (DEI)
1.2. Are there laws and/or regulations on education and training?	at national level	at national level	at national level
1.3 Supervisory authority for nurses' education and training	Ministry of Education	Ministry of Education and Science	Ministry of Health
II. 2.1 Training establishments Number of institutions 2.2 Where based	22 institutions non-university institutions - further education establishments	96 university	349 university: 1, lycées: 2, hospitals: 346
2.3 Level at which diploma recognized	Bachelor level	university level	level III - same level as university studies
III. 3.1 Admission requirements Access to nurse's education and training age: previous schooling qualification entrance exam:	no age requirement 12 years written study aptitude test for those with less than 12 years of schooling	12 years secondary education selection on the basis of past marks	17 12 years baccalauréat general knowledge test, psychological tests, interview
3.2 Access to university age: previous schooling qualification: entrance exam:	no age requirement 12 years depends on line of study centralised system	entrance on basis of written test average of previous marks	no requirement 12 years baccalauréat no
3.3 Is there a numerus clausus for nurses? according to what criteria?	yes, the Government and County Council assess local need	yes, set by the University Council according to resources available	yes, set by Health Ministry according to needs of the population in the different regions
IV. 4.1 System for monitoring the quality of education and training Is there a system for monitoring the quality of education and training?	yes	no	yes by Health Ministry
4.2 How does this work? How often? According to what criteria?	The Ministry of Education is represented on examining boards participation in examinations at the end of each of the 3 parts of the nursing education	no	Regional and departmental directorates for health and social affairs, by among others the presidency of the Technical Council and by means of monitoring at least twice a year

147

B.	SPECIFIC INFORMATION	DENMARK	SPAIN	FRANCE
I. 1.1	Legislative framework Diploma/qualification	Sygeplejerske (nurse's) diploma	Titulo de Diplomado Universitaria de Enfermeria	State nurse's diploma
II. 2.1	Admission requirements Age: Previous schooling: qualification: entrance exam:	no age limit 12 years written study aptitude test		17 12 years baccalauréat yes
III. 3.1	Education and training Duration: years months: weeks: hours: other:	$3\frac{3}{4}$ years 45 months	3 years 27 months 116 weeks 3 900 hours theory credit = 10 hours	3 years $37\frac{1}{2}$ months 136 weeks of education 4 760 hours
3.2 a)	Course Total number of hours		3 900 hours	4 760 hours
b)	Theoretical/technical training • total number of hours • how subdivided — nursing — basic science — social sciences	1 800 h approx. 600 h approx. 600 h approx.	not possible to specify	2 485 hours 2 240 hours (nursing, basic science and social sciences) + 245 hours (pedagogical follow-up)
c)	Clinical training • total number of hours • how subdivided — general medicine	1. care of persons in good health and persons whose health is at risk: 25% 2. care of persons suffering from an acute or chronic physical or mental illness: 75%	not possible to specify at least 50%	2 275 hours 420 hours
	— general surgery — child care and paediatrics — maternity care — mental health, psychiatry — care of the elderly	at least 20% of clinical training takes place in the social sector or outside the hospital 25% of clinical training during first part 30% of clinical training during second part 45% of clinical training during third part of training		490 hours 70 hours 560 hours 175 hours
	— home care — other			385 hours 210 hours of public health
3.3 3.4.	Subjects not listed in annex Is education and training identical in all establishments?	yes	nursing administration no	yes

148

B.	SPECIFIC INFORMATION	DENMARK	SPAIN	FRANCE
IV. 4.1.	Remuneration Remuneration for trainees — from whom? — how much? — for which courses?	yes State grants DKR 3 600 for the first two periods of clinical training and all the theoretical courses Monthly remuneration paid by the school for the third clinical period (DKR 9 400)	no	yes, establishments where students study, FF 1 125 FF in second and FF 1 350 in third year for optional hospital placements Attribution of a grant for some students (18928 FF/year)
4.2.	Do training establishments subsidise places where students undergo clinical training?	no	no	no
V. 5.1.	Instructors Level of qualification required to run an establishment	nurse with advanced education	Nursing University teacher	DEI (State nurse's diploma), 5 years' experience, diploma in health management, 3 years' teaching experience, concours and adaptation training for work
5.2	Do those running establishments have to be qualified nurses?	yes	University teacher	
5.3	Qualification required for instructors who are nurses?	Diploma from School of Advanced Nursing Education in Aarhus, masters degree in relevant areas	nurse's diploma	DEI (State nurse's diploma), 5 years' experience, diploma in health management, competitive tests
5.4	Is there a set student/instructor ratio?	no	no	no

149

A.	GENERAL INFORMATION	IRELAND	PORTUGAL
I. 1.1	Legislative framework Diploma/qualification	certificate of 'Registered General Nurse'	Diploma do curso superior d'enfermagem (general nursing diploma) Professional tile: Enfermerio Title - academic degree: 'Bacharel' = 3 years of training in secondary education
1.2	Are there laws and/or regulations on education and training?	at national level	Law Decree 480/88 from 23.12.88 Portaria 195/90 from 17.03.90
1.3	Supervisory authority for nurses' education and training	An Bord Altranais	Ministry of Education and Ministry of Health
II. 2.1 2.2 2.3	Training establishments Number of institutions Where based Level at which diploma recognized	19 hospital Registration + academic diploma + optional 4th year leading to a degree	33 higher education - polytechnic
III. 3.1	Admission requirements Access to nurse's education and training age: previous schooling qualification: entrance exam:	 17 12 years 'leaving certificate' no, interview	 no age requirement 12 years 12° year diploma + entrance exam to secondary education yes
3.2	Access to university age: previous schooling: qualification: entrance exam:	 no age limit 12 years 'leaving certificate' no	 no age requirement 12 years 12° year diploma + entrance exam to secondary education yes
3.3	Is there a numerus clausus for nurses? according to what criteria?	yes, set by Department of Health on the basis of manpower statistics	yes criteria set up by secondary education nursing schools
IV. 1.1.	System for monitoring the quality of education and training Is there a system for monitoring the quality of education and training?	yes	yes
1.2.	How does this work? how often? according to what criteria?	Inspections by 'An Bord Altranais' every 5 years or more frequently if necessary and also checking of examination results	schools (by the institutions concerned) Ministry of Health + Ministry of Education, through an analysis of the action plans and the annual activity report

150

B.	SPECIFIC INFORMATION	IRELAND	PORTUGAL
I. 1.1.	Legislative framework diploma/qualification	certificate of 'Registered General Nurse'	Diploma do curso d'enfermagem geral
II.	Admission requirements		
	age:	17	no age limit
	previous schooling:	12 years	12 years
	qualification:	'leaving certificate'	12° year diploma + entrance exam to secondary education
	entrance exam:	no, interview	yes
III. 3.1	Education and training Duration		
	years:	3 years	3 years
	months:	36 months	28 months
	weeks:		120 weeks
	hours:	4 600 h	4 200 h
	other:		
			Diploma do curso d'enfermagem geral'
3.2. a) b)	Course Total number of hours Theoretical/technical training		4 200 h
	• total number of hours	40 weeks (registration) 58 weeks (registration/diploma)	min $\frac{1}{3}$
	• how subdivided — nursing — basic science — social sciences		
c)	Clinical training		
	• total number of hours	76 weeks	min $\frac{1}{2}$
	• how subdivided		
	— general medicine	20 weeks	
	— general surgery	20 weeks	
	— child care and paediatrics	6 weeks	
	— maternity care	2 weeks	
	— mental health/psychiatry	5 weeks	
	— care of the elderly	6 weeks	
	— home care	1 week	
	— other	operating theatres, accident + emergency, outpatients	
3.3	Subjects not listed in the annex	yes	varies from school to school
3.4	Is education and training identical in all establishments?		yes (ministrial decret n° 195 from 17 March 1990)

B. SPECIFIC INFORMATION	IRELAND	PORTUGAL
IV.		
4.1. Remuneration		
Remuneration for trainees	yes	no
— from whom?	by hospitals and schools of nursing	
— how much?	salary (registration)	
— for which courses?	grant (registration/diploma)	
4.2. Do training establishments subsidise places where students undergo clinical training?	no	no
V. Instructors		
5.1 Level of qualification required to run an establishment	registration in the nurse tutors division of the register	nurse + specialisation in teaching and management
5.2 Do those running establishments have to be qualified nurses?	yes	yes
5.3. Qualification required for instructors who are nurses?	nurse tutor qualification Bachelor Degree from a University	specialist training (licence, specialisation in teaching and management)
5.4. Is there a set student/instructor ratio?	yes, — for theoretical training: 1 tutor for 15 students — for clinical training: variable determined by hospital authorities	yes, 1 instructor for +/- 10 students

A. GENERAL INFORMATION	GREECE		ITALY	
	University degree in Nursing Degree University	diploma in Nursing Technological Educational Institutions	Diploma universitario di Infermiere (university diploma)	Diploma Infirmiere professionale (professional diploma)
I. Legislative framework 1.1. Diploma/qualification				
1.2. Are there laws and/or regulations on education and training?	at national level	at national level	at national and regional level	
1.3. Supervisory authority for nurses' education and training	Ministry of Education	Ministry of Education	Ministry for the Universities and Ministry of Health	
II. 2.1. Training establishments Number of institutions 2.2. Where based	Univ. + TEI 1 university	Univ. + TEI 9 8 schools of Health professions in TEI	+/-300 (falling) university: +/-20 hospital: +/-350 others: +/-10	
2.3. Level at which diploma recognised	University	Technological level	professional diploma and university diploma	
III. 3.1. Admission requirements Access to nurse's education and training: age: previous schooling: qualification: entrance exam:	no age requirement 12 years 'lyceum certificate' (baccalauréat) yes, national written exam	no age requirement 12 years 'lyceum certificate' (baccalauréat) yes, national written exam	18, no upper limit since 1996 13 years secondary education yes, if number of places limited	
3.2. Access to university: age: previous schooling: qualification: entrance exam:	no age requirement 12 years 'lyceum certificate' (baccalauréat) yes, national written exam	no age requirement 12 years 'lyceum certificate' (baccalauréat) yes, national written exam	18 13 years secondary education yes	
3.3. Is there a numerus clausus for nurses? According to what criteria?	yes, set by the Ministry of Education according to the resources of the training establishments	yes, set by the Ministry of Education according to the resources of the training establishments	yes, each region decides according to need	
IV. System for monitoring the quality of education and training 4.1. Is there a system for monitoring the quality of education and training?	no	no	no, no centralised system, but a representative from the Ministry for Health, the Ministry for Universities and Scientific Research attend the final examination	
4.2. How does this work? how often? according to what criteria?	no	no	A national supervisory body will be set up in the future.	

i 16597941

	GREECE		ITALY	
SPECIFIC INFORMATION	degree in Nursing University	diploma in Nursing Technological Educational Institutions	Diploma universitario di Infermiere	Diploma Infirmiere professionale
B.				
I.				
1.1 Legislative framework Diploma/qualification	degree in Nursing University	diploma in Nursing	Diploma universitario di Infermiere	Diploma Infirmiere professionale
II.				
2.1. Admission requirements				?
age:	no age limit	no age limit	18	
previous schooling:	12 years	12 years	13 years	
qualification:	'lyceum certificate' (baccalauréat)	'lyceum certificate' (baccalauréat)	secondary education	
entrance exam:	yes	yes	yes, if number of places limited	
III.				
3.1. Formation Duration				
years:	4 years	4 years	3 years	3 years
months:		36		
weeks:	144	144		
hours:	5 040 – 5 472 h	4 480 h	4 600 hours	4 600 hours
other	8 terms			
3.2. Course				
(a) Total number of hours	no information	4 800 h	4 600 h	4 600 hours
(b) Theoretical/technical training				
• total number of hours	52%			1 750 hours
• how subdivided				
—nursing	22%	955 h	850 h	
—basic sciences	30%	1 080 h	1 350 h	
—social sciences				
(c) Clinical training				
• total number of hours	no information	2 220 h	2 400 h	2 850 hours (including approx. 400 hours of nursing)
• how subdivided				
—general medicine		270 h	+/-500 h	
—general surgery		195 h	+/-100 h	
—child care and paediatrics		180 h	+/-30 h	
—maternity care		75 h	+/-30 h	
—mental health, psychiatry		150 h	+/-30 h	
—care of the elderly		75 h	+/-75 h	
—home care		75 h	+/-50 h	
3.3. Subjects not listed in annex	data processing, research methodology, statistics, health economics	data processing, research methodology	biochemistry, histology, medical techniques	
3.4. Is education and training identical in all establishments?	yes, there may be slight differences	yes, there may be slight differences	yes, but some small room for manoeuvre is left to each university	

B.	SPECIFIC INFORMATION	GREECE		ITALY
IV. 4.1.	Remuneration Remuneration for trainees	no	yes	yes, there is a variable contribution from the regional authorities
	—from whom? —how much? —for which courses?		Ministry of Health DR 60 000 per month during 8th term	
4.2.	Do training establishments subsidise places where students undergo clinical training?	no	no	
			subject under negotiation	
V. 5.1.	Instructors Level of qualification required to run an establishment?	professor or associate professor	professor or associate professor of technical education	?
				Nurse with a special two-year university qualification
5.2.	Do those running establishments have to be qualified nurses?	no	yes, under the law, but not always in practice	?
				Yes, specified university qualification required since 1982
5.3.	Qualification required for instructors who are nurses?	professor, associate professor, assistant professor, lecturer	the same qualification as for other technological education professors	
5.4.	Is there a set student/instructor ratio?	no	no	no

Source: **Ms. Kathleen Keane, Former Chief Education Officer, (Retired) An Bord Altranais.**